Family-Focused Pediatrics

Interviewing Techniques and Other Strategies to Help Families Resolve Their Interactive and Emotional Problems

A Clinical and Teaching Manual for All Pediatric Care Professionals

2nd Edition

William Lord Coleman, MD, FAAP

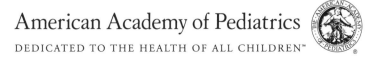

American Academy of Pediatrics

DEDICATED TO THE HEALTH OF ALL CHILDREN™

Published by the American Academy of Pediatrics, 141 Northwest Point Blvd, Elk Grove Village, IL 60007-1098

Library of Congress Control Number: 2011901804
ISBN: 978-1-58110-315-1
MA0459

The recommendations in this publication do not indicate an exclusive course of treatment or serve as a standard of medical care. Variations, taking into account individual circumstances, may be appropriate.

Statements and opinions expressed are those of the author and not necessarily those of the American Academy of Pediatrics.

9-296/0511

1 2 3 4 5 6 7 8 9 10

DEDICATION

In Memory of

Justin Lord Coleman (1976–2003)

Julius Benjamin Richmond, MD, FAAP (1916–2008)

Melvin David Levine, MD (1940–2011)

William I. Cohen, MD, FAAP (1947–2009)

TABLE OF CONTENTS

Section C. Clinical Applications: Techniques for Successful Family Interviewing

Section D. The Family Interview: A Detailed Description

Section E. Conceptual Models of Family Interviewing With Case Studies

Foreword to the Second Edition

*T*he family is the focus, was always the focus, and will always be the
focus for all health care clinicians who take care of children. Dr William
Lord Coleman, a developmental and family-centered pediatrician, and
former member and chairperson of the American Academy of Pediatrics
Committee on Psychosocial Aspects of Child and Family Health, has taken
his passion for children and families to a new level. Prior to the first edition
of *Family-Focused Pediatrics,* year in and year out Dr Coleman would present
his one-person workshop at national meetings. There, he would interview a
family with a particular challenge centered on their offspring in front of an
audience of up to 200 pediatricians using a live video presentation. The family
was shielded from the audience. In this interview, Dr Coleman would quickly
establish the nature of the concern with all family members present and facilitate a conversation of each of the family members' perspectives using a combination of motivational interviewing, psychosocial empathy, compassion,
and his knowledge and integration of family systems functioning and theory.
At the end of the interview (no more than 1 hour), the presenting problems
would be addressed and the family would be committed to an action plan,
which they promised to carry out.

Dr Coleman's first edition addressed how you do it in a very practical
way. This second edition expands on his seminal work. The subtitles of this
superb book are Interviewing Techniques and Other Strategies to Help
Families Resolve Their Interactive and Emotional Problems and A Clinical
and Teaching Manual for All Pediatric Professionals.

In this edition, Dr Coleman takes the reader through concrete steps
and many examples of ways to address the family system as it impacts
on the health of the pediatric patient. He gives us "scripts" and specific
language to use to help us manage those complex problems that can
be effectively addressed in a pediatric setting and do take time.

Some of the clinical scenarios, richly described in detail include
- The son who is always fighting
- Bullying in school
- A 4-year-old girl with temper tantrums
- The "terrific twos" versus the "terrible twos" and parents who cannot set limits
- A 9-year-old girl with chronic abdominal pain
- A tired mother who slaps her son in the office
- A 14-year-old boy with attention-deficit/hyperactivity disorder
- The angry hostile parents
- Marital conflicts
- The 12-year-old girl who is always "depressed"
- The 16-year-old boy who wishes for more positive feedback from his parents

Dr Coleman makes the case for the clinician, interested in behavior and social-emotional family issues, to make a commitment to a special family meeting to see if there can be the beginning of a solution that all family members can agree to. In each case we see the "Coleman model" (brief solution-oriented model) in action. Dr Coleman weaves into his text the family therapy systems theories of Virginia Satir, Salvador Minuchen, and Jay Haley, the great family therapy clinicians and theoreticians. He is clear diagnostically in differentiating child-centered problems and family-centered problems. He takes the clinician step by step into the realm of the family meeting, the goals, the process, and the expected outcome, as one way to address social–emotional concerns. Dr Lynn Wegner also contributes a chapter on payment to legitimize the clinician's time.

One goal of clinicians caring for children is to assess developmental, behavioral, psychosocial, emotional, and family issues. All clinicians, in their long-term, committed relationships with children and families, excel at this. The question is what to do about it once one senses that there are issues or concerns. The clinician at this point has a few options: (1) explore very quickly with the child and parent what the issues are and refer to a mental health or developmental-behavioral clinician, preferable in a collaborative practice with the child or family clinician; (2) identify the concern, and (3) with Dr Coleman's wonderful book as a guide, use some sequestered time, probably no more than a few sessions, to bring the family together to explore options and push for "getting to yes." The clinician should bill for all of these sessions. If a few sessions do not work or if the clinician, in the first session or subsequent sessions, diagnoses complicated psychiatric and family mental health concerns, referral is in order. He tells how to do that, which is also a complicated skill.

For those clinician's interested in common social–emotional issues of children growing up in families, this book reinforces why many of us like taking care of children and families and reinvigorates us to continue this work with his excellent guidance.

Benjamin Siegel, MD, FAAP
Professor of Pediatrics and
*   Psychiatry, Boston University*
*   School of Medicine*
Chair of the American Academy
*   of Pediatrics Committee on*
*   Psychosocial Aspects of Child*
*   and Family Health, 2009–2012*

Foreword to the First Edition

*T*his remarkable, far-reaching book breaks new ground in pediatrics. It is especially useful for behavioral and interactional problems that persist or recur despite traditional child-centered interventions. Dr Coleman's watchword of "your family is your greatest resource" comes alive on every page.

The reader can learn some of the following skills from this book:

- Identifying interactional problems
- Making the shift from child-focused to family-focused intervention
- Facilitating family meetings and family communication
- Helping families rediscover love, respect, communication, and fair play
- Helping families work together, find solutions, and become a team
- Charging appropriately for these services

This book also gives numerous examples of therapeutic strategies and family interviewing techniques as practical illustrations of the skill or skills that it has just taught.

Applying this book to clinical practice should bring the following results:

- An increased comfort level with family disagreements and parent problems
- Rediscovery of the power of words
- Increased creativity in interventions
- Improved ability to help families find and use their strengths
- Doubled therapeutic impact
- Increased personal job satisfaction

No matter what the reader's role in medicine or how much counseling he or she provides, this book helps the reader accomplish it more effectively. The family counseling model crosses many disciplines, giving this book immense value to all clinicians who work with children and adolescents, including general pediatricians, family medicine physicians, developmental-behavioral pediatricians, adolescent medicine specialists, physician assistants, nurse practitioners, physicians and nurses in training, clinical psychologists, social workers, and academic clinical faculty. This practical and timely book gives them methods for taking their skills to a higher level or for teaching those skills to others. This book is for the reader who loves behavioral pediatrics and who wants to learn more about the art and science behind it.

Barton D. Schmitt, MD, FAAP

Preface to the Second Edition

*T*his second edition is intended for all types of pediatric care professionals (PCPs) who care and advocate for children, adolescents, and their families.

It has been reorganized and edited, and includes 2 new chapters: one containing brief descriptions of selected conceptual models of family interviewing and the other explaining the use of procedural and diagnostic codes to document family-focused pediatric care. It serves as both a clinical guide and an informal teaching manual. As a clinical guide, specific family interviewing concepts and other techniques are described and illustrated through many case studies. The American Academy of Pediatrics (AAP) recognized the importance of considering the family in the care and advocacy for children. It concludes, "Children's outcomes—their physical and emotional health and their cognitive and social functioning—strongly influence how well their families function. There is much that practicing pediatricians can do to help nurture and support families and, thus, promote optimal family functioning and children's outcomes....To provide appropriate care for children pediatricians must expand their practices to encompass the assessment of family relationships, health, and behaviors....Families need more support than even the best intentioned pediatrician can provide. Pediatricians are expected by society to advocate for children and families" (AAP Task Force on the Family. *Pediatrics*. 2003;111:1572–1587; AAP Task Force on Mental Health. 2010;125:S87–S108).

Another groundbreaking recent article provides further evidence for the need for a more "family-friendly" pediatric primary care model. "In this qualitative study, pediatric clinicians reflect on the most important elements of high-quality, comprehensive well-child care. Their experience and ideas support a vision of pediatric preventive care that is comprehensive, family-centered, and developmentally relevant, both for children with greatest risk to long-term healthy development and for families with more normative child-rearing concerns. Recent parent focus group findings support these clinician-generated goals in many respects" (Tanner JL, et al. *Pediatrics.* 2009;124:858–865).

This second edition is enhanced by an invaluable chapter on coding and reimbursement by Lynn Wegner, MD, FAAP, entitled "Correct Use of Procedural and Diagnostic Codes to Document Family-Focused Pediatric Care." This chapter offers many suggestions as to how the pediatrician can be reimbursed for practicing family-focused pediatrics.

This second edition will assist PCPs to help children and adolescents and their families resolve their interactive and emotional problems in a more effective, time-efficient, and enduring manner. It will also serve as a clinical teaching guide. A "skills checklist" concludes each section to serve as a teaching guideline.

William Lord Coleman, MD, FAAP
Professor Emeritus of Pediatrics
University of North Carolina
Chapel Hill, NC
Adjunct Assistant Clinical
Professor of Pediatrics
Duke University Medical Center
Durham, NC
November 2010

Preface to the First Edition

There is no perfect child. There is no perfect parent. There is no perfect family. Every family needs help at some time. When they do, they often turn first to the clinician.

Helping children and adolescents with behavioral and interactional problems is one of the great joys and challenges for all clinicians who care for children. Although many of these problems can be solved with an approach that focuses on the child's symptoms, others prove more resistant. When those problems recur or intensify, the clinician should consider an approach that incorporates the family context. This approach, based on the biopsychosocial model, both assesses the child's problem and develops solutions within the family–social context. However, the family counseling skills needed to use this approach are either infrequently or inadequately taught in training programs or continuing education courses.

> *Give a man a fish and he can feed himself for a day. Teach a man to fish and he can feed himself for a lifetime.*
>
> *Chinese Proverb*

Family counseling is effective and efficient because it supports the family, which is the child's greatest resource, and empowers the family to use its own strengths. In using this type of counseling, the clinician not only helps the family resolve the problem but also uses strategies that are more time-efficient and cost-effective. The clinician derives great satisfaction from knowing that the family has developed its own problem-solving techniques (with guidance from the clinician) that will help it not only now but also in the future. Finally, using a family context approach to child care provides the clinician with new intellectual challenges, stimulating him or her personally and revitalizing his or her career.

Teach thy tongue to say, 'I don't know,' and thou shalt progress.
Maimonides

This manual is for clinicians and trainees who want to enhance their skills in working with children and adolescents within the context of their families. These clinicians include pediatricians, family practitioners, pediatric nurse practitioners, child psychologists, child psychiatrists, social workers, and school counselors. It is a beginner's guide intended for those just learning to use a family context approach to resolve behavioral and interactional problems. It is not a textbook on family therapy. This manual describes brief, practical, step-by-step methods for family counseling that the busy clinician can readily incorporate into primary care and can easily tailor for his or her own use. The methods and techniques are liberally illustrated with real-life case studies.

Clinicians work hard because of their deep commitment to improving children's health and well-being, but they must be paid for their effort and time. Therefore, methods for coding and documenting to ensure adequate reimbursement are explained.

After reading this book, the clinician will know how to do the following:
- Identify problems suitable for family counseling.
- Plan family meetings in the office.
- Interview families using a family systems approach.
- Assess family interactions.
- Help families cooperate and develop adaptive behaviors.
- Support parents.
- Improve family communication.
- Deal with disappointments, failures, and difficult families.
- Suggest strategies for specific problems.
- Make a mental health referral.
- Code and document for reimbursement.

The family is the most central and enduring influence on every child. Thus sometimes the best way to help a child is to help the parents. The family context is the domain of clinicians, who have been sanctioned by society to advocate for the child and the family. Family-focused care both satisfies this obligation and fulfills the clinician.

William Lord Coleman, MD, FAAP
Professor of Pediatrics
University of North Carolina

Acknowledgments

D. Anthony Barcel
Whose countless hours and invaluable contributions in assisting me in preparing this second edition are deeply and gratefully appreciated. He is entering medical school in August 2010. He will be a most compassionate, caring, and competent physician with a family focus.

John J. Delaney
Whose remarkable dedication in helping me complete this edition is also deeply and gratefully appreciated. He typed and edited many drafts with great attention to detail and an impressive work ethic. He is entering medical school in August 2011. He too will be a most caring and competent physician with a family focus.

I owe a debt of gratitude to Benjamin Siegal, MD, FAAP, and Greg Prazar, MD, FAAP, for their very useful editing help. I also want to acknowledge the very helpful comments of Barbara Howard, MD, FAAP; Lane Tanner, MD, FAAP; and Larry Wissow, MD, FAAP, FAACAP.

Lynn M. Wegner, MD, FAAP, has written an indispensable chapter on coding and payment ("Correct Use of Procedural and Diagnostic Codes to Document Family-Focused Pediatric Care"). Clinicians must be paid for their services, and family-focused care presents even more of a challenge for payment. Dr Wegner's chapter will prove very helpful to every clinician. I appreciate her effort very much.

The Child, the Family, and the Pediatric Care Professional

Chapter 1

Who Should Read This Book

- Have you ever thought if you could only help a child's family, the child would be better?
- Have you ever experienced clinical frustration, fatigue, and confusion because your well-intended, child-focused therapeutic efforts didn't work anymore and/or the child's and family's problems were worsening?
- Have you ever wondered why parents won't or can't follow your advice or adhere in other ways?
- Have you experienced the gratification of helping a child and family resolve their emotional and relationship issues?
- Have you ever wished you had a clinical guide to help you?
- Have you ever wished you had a teaching manual to help students, trainees, and residents learn family interviewing skills?

This book, intended for both clinicians and trainees, will help you with these challenges. It is not a textbook on family therapy. It is a clinical guide and teaching manual. As a clinical guide it is intended for all those pediatric care professionals who care for, counsel, and advocate for children, adolescents, and their families. These include physicians, psychiatrists, nurses, nurse practitioners, psychiatric nurse practitioners, psychologists, clinical social workers, teachers, counselors, and clergy.

This book is a guide intended for both those just learning a family context approach for behavioral and interactional problems and for experienced professionals. It describes brief, practical, step-by-step methods for family-centered care that can readily be incorporated into any encounter with a child and his or her parent(s). The methods and techniques are illustrated with many real-life case studies.

Each chapter serves as a teaching module with guidance from the teacher, preceptor, or mentor. While not a specific teaching manual per se, its format allows it to be a teaching manual; each chapter offers many specific skills that serve as teaching points. It will serve a variety of trainees and students, including those in the following fields: medical school; nursing; social work; clinical psychology; residents; doctoral students; and fellows in developmental and behavioral pediatrics, adolescent medicine, and child psychiatry.

It is for those who want to provide a family-oriented approach to the evaluation and treatment of a variety of behavioral and social–emotional problems within the family context. This approach often provides more cost-effective and longer lasting results than the traditional child-centered biomedical focus alone.

Chapter 2

Qualifications of the Pediatric Care Professional to Work at the Family Level

*T*he pediatric care professional (PCP) is qualified to use a family approach because of his or her special long-standing trust and relationship with the family. The PCP knows and understands the family and the child, and also trusts them to work together for the benefit of all. The family in turn knows the PCP understands them, cares about them, and is knowledgeable. They trust the PCP to help them. This special relationship allows the PCP to treat a child's issue (eg, depression or a behavioral concern) within the family context. The PCP joins with the family to resolve the issues.

Parents expect PCPs to work with them on issues such as discipline, divorce, sibling interaction, and emotional health, as well as the parents' concerns about their children's development. Sometimes the best way to help a child is to help the parents. Parents expect PCPs to help them with their own personal issues, and PCPs also believe they should help the parents and/ or make referrals.

Some qualifications of PCPs are listed in Box 2.1.

Box 2.1. Qualifications of Pediatric Care Professionals (PCPs) to Work at the Family Level

- PCPs are usually the only ones to see a child and interact with the family in the first few years of the child's life.
- PCPs are positioned to detect "predictable" family concerns (eg, the stress of adapting to the new parental roles) as soon as they arise.
- PCPs see the child when the family presents with the child, as the "identified patient" or the "symptomatic patient" of a disturbed family (eg, the child with recurrent somatic complaints whose parents are experiencing marital conflict).
- PCPs have continuing contact with children and their families. They observe changes as they develop over time. They form a trusting and confidential relationship with the family.
- PCPs contribute to parents' understanding of a child's development, behavior, and child–parent relationships. They also help improve family communication.
- PCPs readily employ a family perspective to help families understand their issues, often an admixture of developmental variation/dysfunction, temperamental differences, behavioral and emotional problems, parental problems, perturbed family dynamics, and outside economic and social issues.
- PCPs, with their knowledge of the family's social context, strengths, and weaknesses, know when to shift to a family perspective.
- PCPs provide anticipatory guidance, screening for behavioral and family psychosocial problems, and primary care treatment.
- PCPs are not perceived as mental health professionals, so families often feel more comfortable seeing them. PCPs know when and to whom to refer.
- PCPs are often more available, accessible, and affordable than other specialists.
- PCPs collaborate with other professionals to improve the care of children and families.
- PCPs are sanctioned by society to advocate for children and families. Courts, schools, police, social agencies, religious institutions, and community organizations expect PCPs to help families and look to them for guidance.

Chapter 3

Understanding Family Systems and Resolving Issues Within the Family Context

A family is a group of individuals who live together and who are related biologically, legally, or socially (eg, an unmarried partner of a parent). A family, however, is more than just a group; it is a unit with its own image, including the attendant goals, issues, values, strengths, and attributes. All families have several roles in common. Together they attempt to carry out the multiple responsibilities of family life, such as providing food, clothing, shelter, education, moral values, love, and nurturing. Families share their lives emotionally as they meet the needs of each individual as well as the whole. A family parent may be a mother and father, parent and partner, single parent, foster or adoptive parents, or a relative. Families may be nuclear (biological father and mother), blended, step, gay, lesbian, bisexual, or transgender.

The family system is characterized by its structure and function, both of which define relationships. The family system includes the composition and organization of the family, the hierarchy (power structure), the subunits (eg, parent dyad, siblings), and the family membership (all who live in the home). Each member has a position in the family "power structure." Family function is how the members and the subsystems interact, how they perceive each other, how they communicate, and how they designate roles. The family system maintains the family balance or stability, but it is altered or "unbalanced" when experiencing stress and change. The stressors may include social, economic, changes in family composition, diagnoses of illnesses, and environmental issues; others are crime, terrorism, and war/deployment (effects on adults and children). The family's challenge, whether transient or permanent, is to adapt to the new reality.

Clinicians are familiar with the organ systems perspective of health and illness. Because illness in one organ affects the whole system, the treatment of a specific organ must take into account its impact on other organs in the system. The clinician must view families with a similar systems perspective: A problem for any member affects every member of the family system.

Family and social factors affect the child, the child's problem/symptom, the parents, and the family interactions. Some family factors are the parents' psychosocial health, their parenting practices and perceptions of the problem, and the family structure and function (hierarchy, roles, relationships). The clinician must consider the impact of these factors on the child and the family and their ability to adapt.

Children cannot be helped in isolation without considering the family context.

Parents of well children need advice, understanding, and support— consider first-time parents, parents adjusting and attaching to a new baby (including paternal and/or maternal depression), early concerns about development and behavior management, prevention efforts of all kinds, making sense of problems with school learning, social success, health and behavior risks in teens, family financial–career stresses, single parents, and divorce. Supporting the child means supporting the parent(s).

Children with acute/chronic illness and/or developmental or intellectual disabilities (in pediatrics by definition dependent for care from their family during times or lifetimes of illness or disability) need comprehensive care that does more than manage the health crisis of the moment. It should also be about building knowledge and skills in the family to handle future problems, and supporting the recovery and development of resilience in the child.

Clinical work may be family-oriented or family-conscious, with or without the full family present (virtual and actual family interviewing). For example, "family awareness" is in evidence when the clinician asks a depressed new mother about her relationship with the child's father, or asks a parent struggling with her preschooler's behavior how her own parents practiced discipline when she was a child.

The family context is the major focus, but equal attention is placed on the child and the family. Pediatric care professionals (PCPs) may shift back and forth between a child focus and a family focus as a way to better understand the problem, but the ultimate focus is the child within the family.

The family is the primary source of many health beliefs and behaviors that affect the child and family. The family's cultural background religious/ spiritual traditions, expectations, and past experiences influence parenting practices.

The PCP cannot fully understand the child–parent relationship by knowing them only as 2 separate individuals. Behavior takes place within a relationship, so PCPs must know the child–parent relationship and gauge the ways in which a change or stress in one affects the other and, indeed, the entire family.

Everything that happens to a family happens to the child and everything that happens to the child happens to the family. The family is the greatest single risk and protective factor for a child. Although many children's problems can be solved with an approach that focuses on the child's symptoms, others prove more resistant. When those problems recur or intensify, the professional should consider an approach that incorporates the family context. This approach, based on the biopsychosocial model, both assesses the child's problem and develops solutions within the family–social context.

Family interviewing is effective and efficient because it explores the family system and its perceptions and coping abilities. It supports the family, which is the child's greatest resource, and empowers the family to use its own strengths in co-constructing solutions with the PCP. In using this type of clinical interviewing, the PCP helps the family resolve the problem with strategies that are more time-efficient, cost-effective, and enduring. However, the family interviewing skills needed to use this approach are either infrequently or inadequately taught in training programs or continuing education courses.

The family interview differs from the traditional patient–clinician interview because it emphasizes understanding the problem within the family–social context and helping the family adapt by developing its own understanding of the family context and mobilizing its resources to work with the PCP.

The interview allows the family and the PCP to appreciate and mobilize their particular strengths and competence of the family (all families have them!) to change the behavior and improve the lives of the family members. Some strengths might be the love and respect of family members for one another, an intact marriage/partnership, their religious beliefs and practices, and their network of support. Focusing on their strengths reduces the inclination of family members to judge or blame each other and instead helps them discover how they have coped thus far and how they are their own greatest resource. Thus the search for strengths is a major component of the interview.

Family systems principles are the basis for a family-oriented approach to behavioral and interaction problems. Making the shift from a focus on the child and the symptoms to a focus on the child within the family context requires knowledge and understanding of family systems principles.

Selected principles and guidelines of family systems and a family context approach are listed in Box 3.1 and brief explanations of these principles and guidelines follow.

Box 3.1. Principles/Guidelines of a Family Context Approach

- Change is inevitable.
- Parents and children influence each other in a reciprocal manner.
- Every family member plays a role.
- Repeating interactive patterns governs family behavior.
- Useful information and observations are obtained by involving the family.
- The family context—child and family—is the major focus.
- The family's health, beliefs, and behaviors affect the child.
- The clinician must understand the child–parent relationship, not as 2 separate individuals.
- Presenting complaints often serve as adaptive or maladaptive functions.
- The family's balance is often maintained by perpetuating the child's symptoms.
- The family system is an integration of structure, function, hierarchy, roles, relationships, and other factors.
- The PCP "joins" with the family to form a therapeutic alliance.

- **Change is inevitable, and the family must adapt to it.** Predictable changes include the birth of a child, death of a family member, the need to balance the marital and parental roles, and meeting the developmental needs of an adolescent. Some unpredictable changes are divorce, medical and/or mental illness in any member, or the diagnosis of a developmental disability in a child. Families with children must accommodate their rapidly changing physical, social, and emotional challenges and needs.

- **The well-being of the child is powerfully influenced by the well-being of his or her parents.** Parents and children each affect one another. When a child has an issue, the developmental tasks of the family are complicated and stressed by the extra attention that the child needs. Therefore, families become a valuable resource for support in managing these problems. Involving the family in the assessment and treatment phases ensures its rightful place in the process as well as a better outcome for everyone.

- **Every member plays a role in the family relationships that tend to maintain or resolve an issue.** Pediatric care professionals need to detect strengths in families, nourish them, and use them to resolve issues. Focusing on issues and concerns often causes family members to blame one another for "the problem." Blaming worsens those issues. If the PCP also implies blame, he or she will lose the trust of the family. For instance, if a child with asthma learns that she can get her way by having a tantrum and inducing an asthmatic attack, who is to blame? The child who wheezes? The parent who "rewards" her when she has an attack? Neither is to blame, yet each is involved in resolving this issue.

- **The behavior of families is governed by repeating interactive patterns.** In the above case, the parents naturally become very sensitive and reactive to their daughter's tantrums, but they may have different approaches. The father may want to indulge her, but the mother may want a firmer approach. While they disagree, argue, and blame each other for "the problems," the girl continues to have tantrums and asthmatic attacks. The family perpetuates "the problem" through its continued interactive patterns. A family systems approach addresses the interactive influences of the girl's learned manipulative behavior, her asthma, and the parents' differing perceptions and responses, and helps implement a healthier interactive pattern.

- **Involving the family in the care of a child provides the clinician with**
  - Information not available from the index patient. Every family member has valuable information, perceptions, and insights that enhance the clinician's understanding of the child and the presenting issue.
  - The opportunity to observe family interactions. Understanding how family members communicate and interact is key to understanding the child and the family.
  - The opportunity to involve the family in the treatment. Helping family members cooperate and develop their solutions (drawing on their own resources, seeking individual and family help, and using social supports) is best accomplished, at least initially, in the family meetings.
  - If the family members can't or won't cooperate in the meeting, they won't do it at home.

- **The family context is the major focus, but equal attention is placed on the child and the family.** Pediatric care professionals may shift back and forth between a child focus and a family focus as a way to better understand the problem, but the ultimate focus is the child within the family. The PCP may focus first on the biomedical aspects of the child's problem (child-centered interviewing), which may include measures such as prescribing medication for a child with attention-deficit/hyperactivity disorder. The clinician then addresses family issues that are affecting the problem (family-centered interviewing), including conflicting parenting practices, differing perceptions of the problem, economic or environmental factors, or stressful career demands on the parent(s).

- **The family is the primary source of many health beliefs and behaviors that affect the child and family.** The family's cultural background, traditions, expectations, and past experiences influence parenting practices.

- **The clinician cannot fully understand the child–parent relationship by knowing them only as 2 separate individuals.** Clinicians usually focus on individual patients. However, because behavior takes place within a relationship, according to the family-oriented approach, they must know the child–parent relationship and gauge the ways in which a change or stress in one affects the other and, indeed, the entire family.
- **Presenting complaints (physical, psychosocial) often serve an adaptive or maladaptive function.** The complaints, maintained by the family, enhance or limit effective family functioning. The child's problem may serve a parent's or the family's need. For instance, a parent who is depressed may focus on a child's issue and maintain it in order to avoid confronting his or her own depression. The child's issue is also the family's issue, because the family is the social group most immediately affected by the child's issue and the treatment. When the child has an issue, the family is in pain. For example, the stress that a child and family feel when going through developmental transitions (either of the child or family) can manifest as somatic, behavioral, and emotional symptoms. These symptoms serve adaptive functions within the family, which then maintains them by its repeating patterns of interaction.
- **The family's balance is maintained by perpetuating the child's symptom.** Families sometimes keep their balance or homeostasis by maintaining the very symptom that brought them to the clinician. For example, a child has recurrent abdominal pain; maintaining the symptom fulfills a parent's emotional need, role, and place in the family and thus maintains the family balance, so the family perpetuates it with its behavior.
- **The family is a system of structure, function, hierarchy, roles, and relationships.** It is also defined by religious, cultural, social, and economic forces. Interactive and communication patterns also characterize the family. The PCP needs to understand a family's particular system and work with the members to define its issues and goals and to develop solutions.
- **The clinician "joins" with the family and forms a therapeutic alliance.** He or she is seen as "a part of" rather than "apart from" the treatment plan. The family's presence and openness are acknowledgments that they need help. The members invite the PCP to enter their family system to help them change a situation that is causing them pain. Joining with the family is similar to forming a therapeutic alliance but implies being a part of the family and not separate from it.

The Family System: A Mobile as a Metaphor

A mobile helps to understand family systems as illustrated in Figure 4.1.

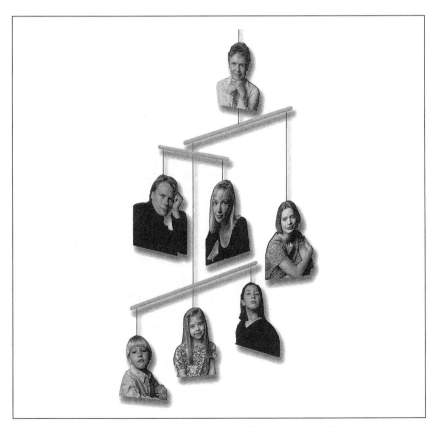

Figure 4.1. The mobile as a metaphor of the family system and its need to maintain balance.

Every member can be positioned and connected in a way that illustrates the structure, hierarchy, relationships, and function of their family system. In this particular mobile (family), the mother is at the top of the hierarchy, and the father is just below her but is slightly above (or at the same level of) his eldest daughter. A second daughter is just below the eldest daughter. Below them, illustrating descending power, are 2 more daughters and a son. Each member has a particular relationship with every other member (ie, emotional and physical distance and closeness). The interpersonal relationships are created and maintained by each member's behaviors, roles, expectations, self-image, position in the hierarchy, boundaries, relationships, and perceptions of others. Like the mobile, the family is in constant motion. Each member's movement contributes to the family movement. Some members move more than others, some are affected by the movement more than others, but all are affected. The whole family works together to balance the system, maintain homeostasis, and help family members maintain healthy and appropriate relationships.

Family systems concepts can be difficult to understand. Also, each family has its unique family system aspects. A visual illustration can be very helpful to the pediatric care professional (PCP), the student, and even to the family. The mobile can also illustrate how a family attempts to maintain "balance" when stressed.

Everything that happens to a child or other family member occurs, at some level, within "the family mobile" and affects all other family members. Everything that affects the family affects the child, like the ripple effect of a pebble dropped in a pond.

Now, blow on the mobile—imagine that this is a breeze (ie, a stress, demand, change) suddenly striking it, causing the mobile to move about and temporarily lose its balance. As the breeze subsides, the mobile quiets and regains its balance. The breeze is a metaphor for the normal transitions and problems that all families encounter. For example, all families face normal developmental transitions (eg, marriage, birth of first child, onset of adolescence, children leaving home, parents at midlife, retirement, and growing older). Any acute psychosocial stress on the family affects the physical, emotional, and social health of each family member. This stress may be temporary and self-resolving or, with the guidance of its clinician, the family resolves the problem. The clinician may also provide directives and interventions (eg, advice, medication, and/or referral).

Now attach a paper clip to one of the figures on the mobile and imagine it as a significant stress or burden on that family member (eg, the diagnosis of a serious medical illness, a changed relationship, or the loss of a parent's job). Notice the change in structure and relationships: some members are grouped closer to the affected member; others become more distant. The hierarchy itself is different. If the problem is resolved, the family mobile regains its balance and resumes its original configuration. However, if the problem is not resolved or if it is only partially alleviated, the family needs to adapt in order to cope with its new reality, represented by the new configuration of the mobile, which is the family's new structure and function.

SECTION A SUMMARY

This section has defined "family" as a social unit that provides care, guidance, learning, values, and protection for a child. There is no one standard or typical family. The family context perspective or family systems approach assesses and resolves a child's issues within the context of the family. The PCP must consider the family structure and function and other various factors, such as position in the hierarchy, roles, expectations, temperamental differences, and beliefs. The interactive behavioral patterns between children and parents must be considered also.

This section also has provided an introduction to family interviewing: purpose, rationale, and benefits of family interviewing; appropriate professionals to treat children within the family context; the unique qualifications of the PCP; the evaluation of a variety of problems and developing solutions within the family context; the benefits of family interviewing; and a family systems perspective.

A mobile has been used as a metaphor for the family. The mobile demonstrates hierarchy, closeness, and distance of family members, and can be used to discuss roles and expectations. The mobile also demonstrates how a minor or major stress or change affects the "balance" and structure altering relationships and roles. The family attempts to regain this "balance" but often needs the help of the PCP to adapt to the new reality.

Skills Checklist

Discuss
- The definition of family
- The concepts of family structure and function
- The necessity for the PCP to understand a family's particular roles, relationships, values, and communication patterns
- The necessity to view the child within the family context
- The importance of focusing on the family's strengths and goals, and the ability to adapt, cope, and develop solutions with their family
- The importance of the PCP in "joining with the family"
- Using a mobile to discuss family structure and function, and the concept of "balance"

Suggested Reading

Allmond BW, Tanner JL. *The Family Is the Patient.* 2nd ed. Baltimore, MD: Williams & Wilkins; 1999

American Academy of Pediatrics. Family pediatrics: Task Force on the Family. *Pediatrics.* 2003;111:1541–1571

American Academy of Pediatrics Committee on Psychosocial Aspects of Child and Family Health. The pediatrician and the "new morbidity." *Pediatrics.* 1993;92:731–733

American Academy of Pediatrics Task Force on Mental Health. The future of pediatrics: mental health competencies for pediatric primary care. *Pediatrics.* 2010;124:410–421

Brazelton TB. Working with families. Opportunities for early intervention. *Pediatr Clin North Am.* 1995;42:1–9

Cohen WI, Milberg L. The behavioral pediatrics consultation: teaching residents to think systemically in managing behavioral pediatrics problems. *Fam Syst Health.* 1992;10:169–179

Coleman WL. Family-focused pediatrics: a primary care family systems approach to psychosocial problems. *Curr Probl Pediatr Adolesc Health Care.* 2002;32:260–305

Combrinck-Graham L. *Children in Family Contexts.* New York, NY: Guilford Press; 1989

Dixon SD, Stein MT. *Encounters with Children. Pediatric Behavior and Development.* 4th ed. Philadelphia, PA: Mosby; 2006

Olson LM, Tanner L, Stein M, et al. Well-child care: looking back, looking forward. *Pediatr Ann.* 2008;37(3):143–151

Schor EL. The future pediatrician: promoting children's health and development. *J Pediatr.* 2007;151(5 suppl):S11–S16

Schor EL. Rethinking well-child care. *Pediatrics.* 2004;114(1):210–216

Tanner JL, Stein MT, Olson LM, Frintner MP, Radecki L. Reflections on well-child care practice: a national study of pediatric clinicians. *Pediatrics.* 2009;124:849–857

Wissow LS, Larson SM, Roter D, et al. Longitudinal care improves disclosure of psychosocial information. *Arch Pediatr Adolesc Med.* 2003;157(5):419–424

Clinical Applications: Preparing for a Family Visit

Chapter 5

Concerns Suitable for Family Interviewing

---

*P*ediatric care professionals (PCPs) encounter many child-centered issues
that eventually will require a family-centered approach. Child-centered
issues are those that the clinician can usually manage with a traditional
child-/symptom-centered approach. These problems generally do not require
a family-oriented approach even though, ideally, clinicians should carry out a
minimal family assessment (eg, family and social histories) for all behavioral
problems. The family with these problems usually responds appropriately to
the clinician's directives. The family is, in general, functionally intact and is
capable of problem-solving and communicating. It is characterized by understanding, love, and empathy for each other and by resiliency. The parents
have no trouble directing the children because boundaries are clear and the
hierarchy is appropriate. Child-centered problems occur in families that are
competent, caring, and capable of problem-solving. These problems affect the
family even though relationships are healthy and the family is coping. These
problems require a minimal family assessment.

Pediatric care professionals often encounter clinical issues that hint at or
suggest a family approach, but the clinician nevertheless might try a child-
centered approach first. The PCP should be sensitive to clues indicating the
need for a family approach: issues intensify or recur despite child-centered
approaches; issues involve changes in family structure and function, and
disturbances in the family system; issues in which parents lack control (eg,
difficulty in establishing or enforcing rules, rewarding good behavior, or dis-
tinguishing inappropriate behavior); and communication problems that strain
family interactions and lead to increasing behavioral and emotional problems
that further disrupt the family.

These issues initially may have been evaluated and managed with a traditional child–symptom approach (eg, generic advice, medication, explanations, and reassurance). These disturbances affect 1 or 2 domains of the child's functioning, such as physical health, school performance, peer interactions, family relationships, emotional well-being, and feelings of security and self-esteem.

Clues suggesting the need for a family-centered approach are listed in Box 5.1.

Box 5.1. Clues Indicating a Family-Centered Approach

- The clinician, working exclusively at the biomedical level, ignores the family context (eg, parenting practices, parental depression).
- The clinician works too hard, repeats instructions, and experiences frustration and failure.
- The problems recur or intensify despite the clinician's interventions. The family is working too hard, is having difficulty communicating, and/or is disappointed and tired.
- The family is wrongly perceived as dysfunctional, noncompliant, or resistant.
- The parent ignores the clinician's advice (Chapter 6).
- The child presents as the "symptomatic patient" or the "identified patient" of a disturbed or stressed family system (Chapter 6).
- Relationship and interaction problems become more apparent ("We don't get along; we need help.").
- The family is unable to resolve the problem and move forward; they feel "stuck" ("We've tried everything.").
- The clinician is unable to resolve the problem; the clinician feels "stuck" ("I've tried everything.") and needs more information.

Family-centered approaches are often preceded by traditional child-centered approaches that fail to resolve the issues. Concerns or issues suitable for family interviewing are biopsychosocial in nature, and they are characterized by relationship–interactive disturbances that recur or intensify despite traditional symptom-centered therapeutic attempts. These issues or concerns also include the challenges of adapting to and supporting children with developmental disabilities or chronic illnesses.

Various disturbances ripple through the family, affecting one or more domains of the child's functioning, such as physical health, school performance, peer interactions, family relationships, emotional well-being, and feelings of security and self-esteem for all family members. Families experiencing family issues are stressed but they are not necessarily dysfunctional, and they are very responsive to time-limited family counseling. Examples of family-centered concerns are listed in Box 5.2.

Box 5.2. Examples of Family-Centered Concerns[a]

- **Relationship problems:** difficult interactions, "not getting along"
- **Social and emotional complications of attention-deficit/hyperactivity disorder and school learning problems**
- **Family communication problems** that discourage expressions of affection, acceptance, and approval and diminish self-esteem
- **Parenting difficulties:** parent–child conflict and a poor fit between child and parent temperaments
- **Emotional problems:** child is experiencing depression, anger, anxiety, grieving
- **Poor compliance with medical regimens**
- **School refusal/separation anxiety**
- **Chronic somatic complaints**
- **Family life cycle events** that cause significant stress (Chapter 29)
- **Behavior problems:** defiant, aggressive behavior
- **Issues** for gay and lesbian families in a heterosexual world
- **Issues** for step, foster, and adopted children and their families
- **Issues** for single parents and their children
- **The impact of divorce** on children and families
- **Challenges** for parents of children with developmental disabilities/chronic illness and the need for family support

[a]Family-centered concerns may be symptomatic of more severe individual and/or family concerns suitable for referral.

Chapter 6

Detecting the Family-Centered Issue: 3 Clinical Settings, Responding to a Telephone Call, and Coding Considerations

CLINICAL SETTINGS

In daily, routine patient encounters, the clinician often detects the problems that may require a family meeting. The idea for a family meeting often arises from 3 common settings: the well-child visit/doorknob question, a visit scheduled because of a behavioral issue, and a telephone call received from a family member about a behavioral issue.

The Well-Child Visit/Doorknob Question

Imagine that, at the end of a well-child visit, a father spontaneously asks about a family-centered problem that is seemingly unrelated to the purpose of the visit (eg, *"My kids are fighting so much my wife doesn't want to come home until they are in bed. What should we do?"*). This concern, the "doorknob question," is a call for help. It may be a hidden agenda or the real reason for coming. In this example, the parent shows his concern and trust in the clinician by revealing sensitive and important information. The clinician must take advantage of this moment; if ignored, the parent may not ask again, and the problem will certainly intensify.

- **The clinician should sit down with the father, obtain a quick overview of the problem, and acknowledge his concern.** The clinician can say, *"I want to hear what's on your mind. We only have a few minutes now, so we can't address your concerns in depth, but we can arrange a visit as soon as possible."* This and the father's brief reply only take 3 to 5 minutes.
- **After the brief discussion, the clinician shows support and interest by**
  — Personally scheduling the next visit as soon as possible. The clinician can call the receptionist from the office in the presence of the parent and ask for the next available appointment time, or he or she can accompany the parent to the reception area to ensure that an appointment is made

as soon as possible. This also shows the caring side of the pediatric care professional (PCP).

— Checking his or her present schedule. If the next patient is running late or has cancelled, he or she can spend more time with the parent.

— Suggesting to the parent that they follow up by phone in the next few days. The clinician can then schedule an appointment with the appropriate family members.

— Considering a referral if he or she feels that the problem is serious even though it would be based on little information. The PCP must help the parent be open to that suggestion for a referral to succeed (Chapter 31).

The Scheduled Visit for a "Behavior Problem"

If, after using several child-/symptom-centered interventions (eg, time-out, medication) the behavior problem remains unresolved, the parent may make a comment such as, *"I try so hard, but I just can't go on like this,"* which suggests to the clinician the need for a family meeting. He or she can respond by saying, *"You have tried many interventions and worked hard, but things aren't getting better. You have a right to feel discouraged. When parents face this situation, scheduling a family meeting often helps them gain more understanding, support, and information."*

Parents may even make overt pleas for help, such as *"My mother-in-law and I are having very serious disagreements about how to raise my son. My husband takes her side, making me feel very frustrated and ineffective."* The clinician in this situation must avoid the appearance of taking sides with either the mother or the mother-in-law and father. Saying something like, *"It sounds like the family has different opinions. That makes it very hard for everyone. If we had a family meeting, we could try and understand the problems better to help the family work together. It would be essential to include your mother-in-law if you agree and if she would join us."*

The Telephone Call About a Behavioral Problem

Clinicians frequently receive calls from parents that indicate the need for a family meeting. In one example of such a call, a mother might say, *"My husband and I think that our son Robbie is smoking marijuana. His dad confronts him often, and they end up in a shouting match, which I have to break up. I'd like you to see Robbie."* The clinician should avoid either assuming the parent role or offering advice on the phone. An appropriate response might be, *"It sounds like everyone is pretty tense. In this kind of situation, meeting with the whole family to understand all the issues is the most helpful. Meeting with Robbie alone or with Robbie and just one parent wouldn't be enough. The whole family has a lot to offer, so I need all of you here."*

RESPONDING TO A TELEPHONE CALL AND CODING CONSIDERATIONS

Phone calls are time-consuming and are inadequate for a proper preliminary assessment. Most PCPs have an established policy about whether to directly charge patients for telephone calls, as payers are variable in their reimbursement for physician telephone services to patients. Moreover, the physician telephone *Current Procedural Terminology* code is very specific about the timing of the call with respect to face-to-face patient visits. It is advisable, therefore, to keep phone calls brief. This will not only help the clinician avoid the appearance of taking sides and prevent him or her from giving hasty and ill-informed advice (based on information from one member speaking privately to the clinician), but will minimize the potential for nonpaid service. (See Chapter 32 for telephone care codes.)

If there is time to discuss this new topic after the preventive health visit, this additional time may be coded as a separate service from the well-child check. If this additional service included more than 50% of the time as counseling, the appropriate visit level would be chosen using time as the visit code criteria. In this situation, modifier 25 would be appended to the preventive service code to show the additional evaluation and management service was separate and identifiable from the well-child check. (See Chapter 32 for modifier use.)

Chapter 7

Ways to Suggest a Family Meeting and Dos and Don'ts

*T*he clinician suggests a family meeting in a way that does not convey blame or incompetence, but that does communicate support, understanding, and hope. The clinician respectfully and clearly states that the family is affected by the problem, that the family is an important resource, and that the whole family will benefit from a meeting.

The clinician often wonders how to actually state the suggestion for a family meeting so that he or she does not appear intrusive, misguided, or dismissive of the parent's stated complaint. Therefore, when the clinician proposes the meeting, he or she must clearly communicate the shift to a family perspective, while emphasizing the importance of the family as a resource for resolving the problem. To do this, he or she might say, *"A family meeting would be very helpful because its purpose is not to focus on any one person or imply blame. Instead we need to understand the issue better by getting everyone's input. Your family is the best resource for that—everyone has something to offer. We will need everyone's perspectives and cooperation."*

The pediatric care professional (PCP) should keep expectations for the meeting realistic for the family (and for the clinician). For example, the clinician should say, *"I'm going to help you improve the tantrum situation a bit, but it will take some time and work and several visits."*

A mother might imply that she doesn't feel supported by saying, *"My husband works longer hours and then stops at the sports bar for a few drinks with the boys."* The clinician can reply with, *"That must be difficult. I feel I am missing something that would help us all understand the issues. I need to hear what you and the others in the family think. A family meeting would be the best way to start."*

WAYS TO SUGGEST A FAMILY MEETING

- **If the parents' initial complaint is centered on interaction and relationship issues,** the parent might say, *"My son and I are always arguing. We just can't get along; my husband is irritated with us both."* The clinician would respond by saying, *"The family has the best understanding of the issues. When someone has a problem like this, I find that getting information from other family members helps. You all have a lot to offer. The family meeting is the only way to do this."*

- **If child-centered interventions fail and the parents return for more advice, the clinician should review the situation with them.** Did they truly understand the problem and were they able to adhere to the suggestions? Did the parents agree with one another? Did the PCP perceive the issues well enough? The mother indicates that adherence has been difficult by saying, *"We did agree with your ideas, but we just couldn't seem to do them."* The clinician, acknowledging the family's efforts and frustration, says, *"Ms Jones, I appreciate all you have done. You have worked very hard, and yet the issue is getting worse. I share your sense of frustration, and I feel that I don't have enough information. A family meeting is the best way to get a better understanding. It's time for us to stop focusing on Josh alone. It's not enough and it's not working."*

- **If the parents openly state a relationship problem, the clinician should view this as a direct plea for help.** In the course of assessing a problem, especially when parents know and trust the clinician, they often reveal a problem in their relationship. One of the parents might say, *"We never talk to each other."* The clinician could respond with, *"From what you say, everyone seems to be affected. That you have tried is apparent, but now things are getting worse because you don't talk to each other. A family meeting allows us to take a broader look at the family to understand the issue. From my experience, when things get to this point, a family meeting is helpful."*

- **If parents become upset (angry, tearful, frustrated) with each other or with their children in the office,** the clinician should explore the situation. He or she must first reflect their feelings (Always Acknowledge Affect— AAA). These supportive statements also serve as invitations for the parent to share information about the family situation. The clinician might say, *"I can see this is very upsetting to you."* After letting the family respond, the clinician might ask, *"Does this happen at home?"* If the family's answer suggests that it does, the clinician can ask what, if anything, the family has tried and can suggest the family meeting in the following way, *"From what I hear, everyone is feeling pretty upset, and you would like to see things get better. When I see a family issue like this, the best thing to do is to have a family meeting. That way no one is singled out. Everyone will share his or her feelings and thoughts, without being criticized or judged, giving us a much* *better idea of what's going on. Then you can begin to work together. Also, everything that happens here is confidential."*

- **If the clinician feels that he or she does not have enough information and needs to explore the family context,** the clinician should admit that he or she is confused and wants more information. He or she could say, *"I don't have enough information. I need to understand the family and how it is responding. A family meeting gives me information not available from an exclusive focus on one member; it also offers more interventions. I would like to schedule a family meeting."*

DOS AND DON'TS

In addition to the techniques described above, the clinician should keep in mind several other practical tips to help the family understand and accept his or her suggestion. These tips (dos and don'ts) are listed in Box 7.1.

Box 7.1. Dos and Don'ts: Practical Tips for Suggesting a Family Meeting

DOs

- *Do* call the complaint an "issue" or "concern" NOT a "problem."
- *Do* select families carefully. The ideal family is one known from prior visits where a comfortable relationship exists.
- *Do* select issues carefully. Focus only on one, such as tantrums or sleep problems. Do not attempt to solve all of the family's problems.
- *Do* remember that progress will take time and effort. Informing the family of this sets realistic expectations and removes pressure from both the clinician and the family.
- *Do* call the gathering a family meeting, family session, or family visit.
- *Do* state clearly that the purpose of the family meeting is to gather more information and to help the family work together to solve their issue.
- *Do* be direct, positive, and confident about the need and benefit for a family meeting.
- *Do* make sure the purpose of the meeting is clear to the person who will inform the rest of the family of the meeting.
- *Do* emphasize the importance of the whole family attending the meeting, ideally at the first meeting.
- *Do* state that all families need help from time to time.
- *Do* offer to meet with most of the family when others can't or won't attend.
- *Do* provide time for questions after requesting a family meeting.
- *Do* identify the family hierarchy and form an alliance with the family leader.

Continued on page 30

Box 7.1. Dos and Don'ts: Practical Tips for Suggesting a Family Meeting, continued

DOs, continued

- *Do* remember the child does not need to be present at the meeting for a bill to be submitted to an insurer. The meeting would be billed on a time basis as the visit is focused on counseling.

DON'Ts

- *Don't* call the meeting "family therapy." Call it a "family meeting."
- *Don't* wait for a crisis to suggest a family meeting, if possible.
- *Don't* imply that the meeting is to explore all aspects of the family life.
- *Don't* imply that the meeting is to reconstitute the family or to challenge its values.
- *Don't* say that the family meeting is to determine how family dynamics or problems affect the child's problem. Relevant issues will reveal themselves in the meeting.
- *Don't* imply that the family is dysfunctional or incompetent.
- *Don't* accept a family's initial hesitation or reluctance to agree to a meeting.
- *Don't* be unclear, hesitant, or uncertain about the need for a family meeting.
- *Don't* imply that anyone is to blame or is at fault.
- *Don't* imply that you have the answer to the issue and that you plan to give advice.
- *Don't* state or imply you are going to refer the family to a mental health professional. That issue, if necessary, will reveal itself in later family meetings and be addressed then and in an appropriate manner.

Chapter 8

Case Study 8.1: Suggesting a Family Meeting

*K*ate, a 7-year-old girl whom the clinician has followed for 5 years, recently has experienced recurrent abdominal pain. Several physical examinations and various laboratory tests, and even magnetic resonance imaging, during the last month were negative. Kate has stopped participating in after-school sports. Her mother, very worried, keeps asking if "another test" might reveal the cause of the pain. At the latest visit, after another normal physical examination and careful review of all the tests, the clinician feels that she needs to know more of the family context. First, she decides to speak privately with the mother.

Clinician (to mother): *I'd like to speak alone with you for a few minutes.* (When Kate looks alarmed, the clinician reassures her by continuing with the following.) *Kate, all of the examinations and tests have been normal. You are a healthy girl. I just need to speak with your mom alone.* After Kate leaves for the waiting room, the clinician continues by saying, *Ms Martin, I've known Kate for 5 years. As you know, all of the examinations and tests have been normal; it doesn't seem like there is a physical cause for her pain.*

Mother: *Why do you think she has these pains? Is she faking them to get out of sports?*

Clinician (demystifying the phenomenon): *No, I am sure she is not. I feel I know her very well. She has always enjoyed sports and done well. As a clinician, I can tell you that the body and mind are not separate. Each affects the other. This holds true for children and adults. For example, if we are worried about something either inside the family or outside but can't or don't want to talk about it, we may have a headache or muscle tension. Kate might be doing the same with her stomachaches.*

In saying this, the clinician has taken time to educate the parent about the connection between emotional/mental distress and somatic pain, has expanded the inquiry, and has created a family–social context for further questioning about nonmedical issues. She has discussed these issues in a calm, reassuring, gently probing manner.

Mother (somewhat doubtful): *I'm not sure what you mean.*

Clinician (exploring the family context): *I'd like to ask about other things that might affect Kate, such as friends, school, and family. Asking about these things might seem a bit strange, but they are important.*

The clinician just gently expanded the evaluation from a child–medical focus to a family–psychosocial focus as well. She moved away from the clinician's traditional biomedical role while emphasizing her concern for Kate's well-being.

Mother: *Go ahead.*

Clinician: *Have there been any recent stresses at school?*

The clinician has deliberately chosen school, a less-threatening topic than family, to expand the focus of the interview.

Mother: *She is doing well. Her grades are good and her teachers report that she is well behaved. The sports thing is the only change. She has decided not to participate.*

Clinician (still pursuing a less personal issue than the family): *How are things with her friends?*

Mother: *She remains popular and has several good friends. In fact, they want her to join the team again, but Kate refuses.*

The clinician now explores the family situation in a very general but indirect way.

Clinician: *I haven't seen Mr Martin for a long time. What does he think about Kate's stomachaches?*

Mother: *He is so busy at work that he has hardly noticed. He cares, but he knows I am taking good care of Kate.*

Clinician (following up on mother's comment): *I know you are. Is he working more than ever?*

Mother: *Yes, it seems like he is....*

The mother pauses and the clinician remains silent. Silence allows the mother to recognize her own feelings and to share them if she wishes.

Mother: *It seems like he is avoiding us...or me. When I ask for help, he always has an excuse. We argue a lot.*

The clinician now asks a more specific question that follows from the information just offered. This keeps the line of questioning nonthreatening but logically related to the conversation.

Clinician: *Have the arguments been more frequent over the past month or two?*

Mother: *Yes. They get quite unpleasant at times.*

The clinician's questions and the information received have revealed a possible connection between the family stress and the stomachaches and have confirmed the clinician's suspicion. Next, she makes the mother a partner in evaluating the problem within a family context.

Clinician (exploring the parent relationship and the concern): *Do you think that the stresses between you and your husband might be contributing to Kate's stomachaches?*

Mother: *I hadn't thought about that, but now that we have talked I think there is a connection. She does seem worried and spends more time in her room alone. Things at home are tense even if we aren't arguing.*

At this point the clinician can suggest that a family meeting is the next logical and useful step.

Clinician: *A family meeting would be very helpful. It's apparent that there is a lot going on and that everyone is feeling some pain. The meeting would help everyone understand the issues. By working together, you could begin to resolve them. Your family is your greatest resource.*

The mother agrees to discuss the possibility of a meeting with her husband. She will call the clinician next week.

Chapter 9

Who Should Attend a Family Meeting

*I*nitially the pediatric care professional may choose to interview only the most involved family members, after identifying all family members who live in the home. At some point the whole family should attend the meeting. This is especially important for the first meeting. The head of the family must always be in attendance.

If that is not possible or if the family is too large, both parents (or parent figures), the "identified patient," and any other key family member(s) (eg, sibling, grandparent) should attend the meetings. The clinician should insist that both parents attend the meetings; this should not be used as a threat but should emphasize the importance of their input for understanding the problem and of their cooperation for resolving it. Within a single-parent family, the parent might invite another person who either cares for the child or is influential (eg, the parent's partner, another family member, or friend). If a single parent has a partner living in the house, that partner is considered part of the family and should be invited to the family meeting. The clinician should discuss this first with the parent to gain his or her approval.

If only a portion of the family attends, the clinician and the members present at the meeting must decide if the "partial" family meeting has been beneficial. If it has not been, the clinician should ask the family to bring the other members at the next visit. It is critical for all family members to attend the family meeting. If this is not possible, the clinician may have to discontinue family meetings. However, he or she can still follow an individual child and can continue to advocate for that child and make referrals for the family.

Chapter 10

Arranging the Office for a Family Meeting

*H*aving a roomy, comfortable, family-friendly meeting space available for the meeting is an ideal component. The clinician can do 2 things to arrange the office for the interview: find space (an ample, comfortable room) and obtain equipment (toys, paper and crayons, and tissues).

SPACE FOR THE INTERVIEW

Most offices and clinics contain only standard, narrow examining rooms. Although these rooms are not ideal, they can be made more family-friendly if the clinician provides small chairs and cushions for the children. A more suitable space is a room where the chairs can be arranged in a loose semicircle, or circle: a conference room, the clinician's office, or the waiting room if the meeting occurs after regular office hours. If the meeting takes place in the clinician's office, the clinician should not sit behind his or her desk because that arrangement appears too formal and creates a "barrier" between the clinician and the family, discouraging the sense of "joining."

If the parent or clinician wants to discuss something privately, children should leave the room for a while. Parents invariably appreciate this time alone with the clinician. In this situation, children can sit in the hallway, the next room, the waiting area, or the playroom with a book, toy, or drawing material to keep them occupied while they wait. Teenagers appreciate the availability of a separate waiting room especially equipped for adolescents with appropriate age-level reading material.

Examination rooms should have seating for everyone, including the clinician. Standing becomes uncomfortable and can convey to the family a sense of clinician dominance, impatience, or disinterest.

If the family and clinician are seated at a table, an ideal table is a round one because the seating arrangement implies equality. If a round table is not available, seating the parent, who needs to be perceived as the parent in charge, at the head of the table is often helpful. Sometimes, placing no one at the head of the table works best if the family needs to encourage more expression and initiative from some members.

A carpeted room is handy because the floor can be used as a place for the children to draw or play—it might actually be the only place available for this. At times, the clinician might need to sit on the floor with the children to engage them.

EQUIPMENT

Toys and drawing materials to amuse and occupy the children during the visit should be available. More important, they are often useful because they help children express themselves. The clinician should observe the children during play to figure out what the children's actions and words communicate about their feelings. Some children actually can be interviewed better while they are drawing or playing. In addition, a family drawing by the child or hand puppet play can be used to help parents and children interact and communicate. Some suggested supplies include large sheets of paper, crayons, pencils, felt-tip pens, hand puppets, books, and small toys (Chapter 28). A box of tissues should also be kept handy because family meetings often evoke painful feelings.

Chapter 11

Scheduling a Family Meeting

*P*lanning in advance results in an organized and time-efficient meeting. Therefore, the clinician should set a time schedule and then plan the final details in the pre-meeting phase.

SCHEDULING THE SESSIONS

For working parents, family visits usually are most convenient when planned for the late afternoon or early evening. Some clinicians reserve a day or a half-day for behavioral–developmental concerns and family sessions; others have regular weekend office hours. Another option for the clinician is to modify his or her schedule by blocking out more time for a single visit or by scheduling several closely spaced, shorter visits. This willingness to work around the family's schedule is important because finding a convenient time for the family greatly enhances the likelihood of its keeping the appointment. By being flexible with his or her scheduling, the clinician also shows his or her personal commitment to the family.

TIME ALLOTMENT

Depending on the nature of the problems and on how well the clinician knows the family, the initial family meeting generally requires 40 to 50 minutes. For those clinicians who cannot devote that amount of time to one meeting, the initial family meeting can be divided into 2 visits. Follow-up visits usually take 30 minutes.

PRE-MEETING PHASE

In the pre-meeting phase, the clinician should prepare a plan for the interview session. Organizing improves the chance that the upcoming meeting will be time-efficient, productive, and satisfying. Topics to consider in this phase include deciding which people should attend and forming a general hypothesis and plan.

SECTION B SUMMARY

This section has described clinical applications. To guide the pediatric care professional, it has listed, in logical order, concerns suitable for family interviewing, detecting a family issue, ways to suggest a family meeting (switching from a child focus to a family-context focus), a case study illustrating how to suggest who should attend a family meeting, how to arrange the office, and how to schedule a family meeting.

Skills Checklist

Discuss

- Issues suitable for a family-focused interview and what distinguishes them from a child-focused interview
- Clues suggesting the need for a family method
- How to suggest the switch to a family focus
- Who should attend family meetings
- How you might arrange your clinical space to best accommodate a family meeting
- How to plan for sufficient time for the meetings
- Consider your own cases and how you might suggest a family meeting

Suggested Reading

Allmond BW, Tanner JL. *The Family Is the Patient*. 2nd ed. Baltimore, MD: Williams & Wilkins; 1999

Brazelton TB. Working with families. *Pediatr Clin North Am*. 1995;42:1–10

Campbell TL, McDaniel S. Conducting a family interview. In: Lipkin M, Putman SM, Lazare AR, eds. *The Medical Interview*. New York, NY: Springer-Verlag; 1995:178–186

Coleman WL. *Family-Focused Behavioral Pediatrics*. Philadelphia, PA: Lippincott Williams and Wilkins; 2001

Coleman WL. Family-focused pediatrics: a primary care family systems approach to psychosocial problems. *Curr Probl Pediatr Adolesc Health Care*. 2002;32:260–305

Combrinck-Graham L. *Children in Family Contexts*. New York, NY: Guilford Press; 1989

Dodson LS. *Family Counseling, a Systems Approach*. Muncie, IN: Accelerated Development, Inc.; 1977

Doherty WJ, Baird MA. *Family Therapy and Family Medicine*. New York, NY: Guilford Press; 1983

Dixon SD, Stein MT. *Encounters with Children. Pediatric Behavior and Development*. 4th ed. Philadelphia, PA: Mosby; 2006

McDaniel S, Campbell TL, Seaburn DS. *Family-Oriented Medical Care: A Manual for Medical Providers*. New York, NY: Springer-Verlag; 1990

Nichols MP, Schwartz RC. *Family Therapy: Concepts and Methods*. 2nd ed. New York, NY: Allyn and Bacon; 1991

Stuart MR, Lieberman JA. *The Fifteen-Minute Hour: Applied Psychotherapy for the Primary Care Physician.* 2nd ed. Westport, CT: Praeger; 1993

Weber T, McKeever JE, McDaniel SH. A beginner's guide to the problem-oriented first family interview. *Fam Process.* 1985;24:357–364

Clinical Applications: Techniques for Successful Family Interviewing

Chapter 12

Communication Skills

―――――■―――――

*E*ffective communication between the pediatric care professional and the family is at the heart of a productive family meeting; the essence of forming a therapeutic alliance. In the family interview the clinician mostly listens, and the family mostly talks. Several communication skills are described in Box 12.1.

Box 12.1. Communication Skills

- Listening empathetically
- Listening actively
- Ensuring clear communication
- Permitting silence
- Listening without interrupting

LISTENING EMPATHETICALLY

Listening with empathy is the most important skill for the clinician. It can be defined as the ability to listen and to respond to the family's emotions and thoughts with compassion and understanding. Without filtering or judging what the family is saying, the empathetic clinician conveys a genuine interest and respect for the family.

The clinician can develop and convey empathy by reflective listening, which means the clinician acknowledges the family members' feelings and concerns so that they sense that the clinician shares their feelings and does not judge them.

Some examples of responses that the clinician may offer include the following:

- *"That must have been difficult for you."*
- *"You must feel proud of your son."*
- *"You look sad when you mention this topic."*
- *"I don't know how you did it."*

LISTENING ACTIVELY

Active listening is listening and then responding to the family in verbal and nonverbal ways. Verbally, the clinician actively listens by making brief comments every once in a while. He also summarizes, which condenses and clarifies information and assures the speaker that he or she is understood. The clinician should ask if everyone is in agreement. Summarizing can be done at several points in the interview. These mini-summaries also help the family retain information (eg, *"Let me be sure I follow you. You have said that...."*). Nonverbal active listening involves leaning forward slightly, minimizing movement of hands or feet, making appropriate eye contact, and assuming a facial expression and tone of voice that match the happy or sad mood of the family.

ENSURING CLEAR COMMUNICATION

The clinician must be sure that what he or she says to the family, what the family says in response, and what the family says to each other contain no ambiguity or misunderstanding. Accomplishing this improves the clinician's understanding of the family and also helps the family members communicate more clearly and effectively with one another. The following items help ensure clear communication:

- **Avoid medical or technical jargon** (eg, "family dysfunction" or "mood disorders"). These terms often make families feel stigmatized or confused. The family often doesn't understand these terms or misinterprets them to mean that the family is "crazy" or "abnormal."
- **Stay away from dispensing too much information at one time** (eg, talking at length or giving too many details). This overwhelms the family's ability to retain the information or to determine the most important points. It also reduces the available time for the family members to talk, communicate with each other, or ask their own questions.
- **Keep away from speaking too rapidly** (eg, at a fast, pressured pace). Speaking rapidly reduces the family's ability to "follow" the conversation and to remember and understand the information. It also makes the clinician seem hurried and disinterested.

- **Offer to clarify the message for the family.** For example, the clinician might follow a comment with, *"Does this make sense to you?"* or *"Would you like me to repeat it or say it another way?"*
- **Make sure that family members understand each other.** One of the most common family issues is poor communication, even in the clinician's office. The clinician can help the family members communicate better during the family meeting. Asking questions, such as *"Did you understand what your mother said?"* or *"Would you like her to say it again?"* helps clarify misunderstandings.
- **Clarify any vague or subjective words or phrases.** For example, if the speaker uses words like *"lazy,"* *"slow learner,"* or *"not so good,"* the clinician should guarantee that everyone in the room (including the clinician) understands what the speaker is saying by asking questions, such as, *"What do you mean by 'lazy'?"* or *"Can you explain what you mean by 'bad attitude'?"*
- **Encourage elaboration to get a more detailed description of the issue.** For example, respond with, *"Tell me more,"* or *"Describing in more detail would help me and the others to understand better."*
- **Ask the family to specify references to others.** For example, if the speaker says, *"She says...,"* the clinician can ask, *"Who do you mean by 'she'?"*
- **Ask the family to specify behavior.** For example, if a family member says, *"He never does what he's told,"* the clinician asks a question to define that reference, such as, *"What is he told?"* or *"Never?"*

PERMITTING SILENCE

The family interview often evokes strong feelings and thoughts, which can be difficult or painful to discuss. Permitting silence, far from wasting time, allows the family to reflect on its feelings, to organize its thoughts and feelings, and to regain its composure. Silence also provides an opportunity for a quiet or hesitant family member to speak. If the family appears uncomfortable with silence, the clinician should start with brief periods of silence (5–10 seconds) and gradually extend them (15–30 seconds) if they prove appropriate and productive.

LISTENING WITHOUT INTERRUPTING

When the clinician listens without interrupting, he or she helps the family tell its story and conveys respect and interest. Frequent interruptions fragment the interview, frustrate the family, and lessen the chance of gaining important information. A speaker usually pauses spontaneously after talking for about a minute to let the listener respond. At this point, the clinician can ask questions, offer comments, or encourage another member to speak (eg, *"Susan, would you like to respond to your father?"* or [to the speaker or another member] *"What are you feeling now?"*).

SEARCHING FOR STRENGTHS AND PAST SUCCESSES

Talking only or at length about "problems" or concerns can be very discouraging to both the family and the clinician. To add hope, creativity, and energy to the meeting and to gain useful information, the clinician should ask about family strengths and past successes. A discussion of past successes can be used as a basis for constructing more solutions and providing direction and support. For example, *"Ms Garcia, tell us something about Roberto that makes you proud or happy or tell us about a time when you all did something that made you feel good about being a family."*

Chapter 13

Techniques to Facilitate a Successful Family Interview

A family interview differs from a traditional pediatric visit in which the pediatric care professional (PCP) usually interviews the parent about the child's problem. In the family interview, the PCP must communicate simultaneously with the parent and the child, strengthen the child–parent bond, and form strong bonds between the PCP and the parent and child. After brief problem talk, the PCP must help the family clarify their goals and share their perspectives or beliefs about the goal. Nine strategies to facilitate a successful family interview are described below.

COMPLIMENTING THE FAMILY

Compliments express respect for and recognition of the family's efforts, strengths, and commitment to and affection for one another. Giving compliments also models good parenting skills. When the clinician compliments a child in the meeting, he or she is showing the parent how to praise the child for good behavior, thus reinforcing it.

Compliments should be given in the interview as opportunities arise. The entire family can be complimented on past actions or behaviors in the meeting. Even attending the meeting is an achievement that deserves a compliment. The clinician should recognize that parents need and deserve compliments as much as children do.

Compliments can be
- **Verbal** *("Nice job. You're a really hardworking parent.")*
- **Nonverbal** (a smile, nod of the head, a handshake, or a "high five")
- **Note taking** (clinician very deliberately jots a note in the chart while exclaiming, *"Wow, that's impressive!"*)

- **Direct** (giving the compliment directly to the person)
- **Indirect** (asking another member, *"Did you hear that?"* or *"Wasn't that nice?"*)

Giving compliments also ends the interview on a positive note and leaves the family with hope, a sense of competence and accomplishment, and a willingness to return.

REMAINING NEUTRAL/NOT TAKING SIDES

Staying in "the middle of the road" removes the focus (and implied blame) from "the identified patient" (usually the child). It conveys respect for and acceptance of each member's perspective and also eliminates the formation of a coalition between the clinician and a family member. Everyone is then assured that the clinician is working for the family's well-being. This perception of impartiality ("fairness") helps the clinician gain each member's trust and increases their willingness to comply with suggested interventions. Clinicians should be especially vigilant in the following situations:

- Parents who don't agree on discipline
- A parent who feels that he or she has too much responsibility for child care
- A parent who feels unappreciated by his or her spouse/partner
- A disgruntled parent or child who tries to persuade the clinician to take his or her side
- A parent and child who disagree about family rules (eg, curfew hours)

In these situations, the clinician must remain neutral if he or she is to gain the trust and cooperation of all the family members. However, remaining neutral is often not easy. For example, a father who is excessively and unfairly criticized by his in-laws needs the support of the clinician in a way that does not antagonize the in-laws. One way a clinician might accomplish this is to form a stronger alliance between the father and the mother so that they support each other.

CONFRONTING

When the clinician feels that confrontation is the only way or the last chance to gain a more truthful answer, to interpret or resolve an apparent contradiction, or to challenge an assumption, he or she should confront that family member. The clinician can try to determine if a challenge will succeed (eg, get a truthful answer) or if it will backfire (eg, antagonize the member), but often he or she will not know until the challenge actually occurs. It can be done by asking the family member a direct question or by making a statement in a clear, nonjudgmental manner. Below are examples of situations when the clinician might confront a family member or the whole family.

- Emphasize the importance of particular information.

Clinician: *Parent stresses strongly influence children.*

If the parent does not respond then, the clinician may repeat or rephrase the statement/question later in the interview when the parent is more comfortable.

Clinician: *As I said earlier, parents often experience stressful situations that affect their children. Have you experienced any stresses recently that might be affecting your child?*

- Confront generalizations.

Father: *We never have any peace.*

Clinician: *Never? Surely there must have been times when there was some peace.*

- Challenge assumptions.

Mother: *My 3-year-old should know better.*

Clinician: *He should? Tell us what you mean.*

- Resolve an apparent contradiction.

Clinician: *When we spoke on the phone, you were very worried; however, now you appear very happy. I am confused. I need to know how you really feel and what you want.*

- Resolve inconsistencies between feelings and body language or between content and affect.

Clinician: *You're talking about something that is very upsetting, but I can't tell by looking at you. You seem so at ease.*

Clinician: *You are discussing your child's use of bad language, but you don't sound very worried.*

REFRAMING

Reframing is a method used to change the family's incorrect, negative perception of one member's mood or behavior to a positive, more correct perception by explaining or "demystifying" it. The process also gives new meaning to one's own behavior or role in a relationship. For example, a clinician might reframe a "bad" child as one who "has poor impulse control," which is a symptom of his particular type of attention-deficit/hyperactivity disorder. In the same way, an "irritable" or "mean" parent is reinterpreted as a "sad" parent, who is depressed and tired.

NORMALIZING

When a family has a problem, it often thinks that it is the only one with this problem. It labels itself as "abnormal," which only adds to its feelings of stress, shame, or secrecy. The clinician can correct this false impression by normalizing the problem in 1 of 2 ways. One method places the family's problem within the range of normal variation—a common, non-severe problem that is experienced by others. For example, a family makes an appointment with the clinician because the 7-year-old son is experiencing encopresis. Both the parents and child are ashamed. The clinician can allay the boy's worries a bit by saying, *"I take care of many kids with the same problem. It's a common problem, and it's normal to feel embarrassed."*

Another mode of normalizing occurs when parents call because of intense parenting disagreements. The clinician can respond by saying, *"It is normal to feel this intense stress under these conditions. The harmony and stability within families comes and goes. The problem does need attention, but your willingness to seek help is a measure of your ability to cope and restore harmony."* In this instance, normalizing does not mean that this situation is a normal occurrence; however, it does mean that the problem, although severe, is a normal reaction and that the family needs help like all families do at various times.

AVOIDING THE PARENT ROLE

Parents sometimes expect or want the clinician to assume the role of a parent (eg, *"Can you talk some sense into our son?"*). However, the clinician should sidestep this role because it presents several problems.

- The child may perceive the clinician as another parent instead of as a neutral figure. He or she may then reject the clinician's advice.
- The clinician's role is to help the parents cope and adapt, not to convince the child to do something.
- It removes parental authority from the parents when they need to be empowered. Therefore, the child may continue to disobey them.
- The clinician may be perceived as intrusive and paternalistic if he or she acts as a parent without being asked.
- The clinician should instead provide leadership without becoming the parent. Being the "parent" undermines parental authority.
- The clinician should give extra support to the parents, as though he or she were parenting the parents, when they have weak parenting skills. The following examples show how the clinician can do this without usurping parental authority and without being overly directive or obvious.
  — In a meeting, the clinician can excuse the child so that the clinician and parent can have a private talk. This conveys a sense of hierarchy and adult–parental authority to the child. With the child out of the room, the clinician can make suggestions to the parents who then communicate them to the child when he or she rejoins the meeting.

— Sometimes, if a child is disrespectful (swearing at or belittling the parent), the parent is unable to reestablish proper parental authority. In this case, the clinician temporarily forms an alliance with the parent and acts as a coparent to help the parent regain control and establish rules, limits, and consequences. At this point the PCP may excuse the child from the room and give the parents a "script" with which to tell the child that they are in charge and that the clinician supports them. *"It is essential that you regain control and assert your authority. I suggest you tell your child that you are the parents, you are in charge, and you are going to set some rules, and that I am very supportive of the two of you."*

TAKING BRIEF, SELECTIVE NOTES

Clinicians should not take detailed notes, as this "removes" them from the family. Tell the family that you wish to take some notes for your records, but that it is all confidential. In some situations the clinician should not take notes if it might compromise the family's openness or if the family objects. Brief and selective note taking instead can be very useful for the following reasons:

- Selective note taking lets the clinician pay attention and communicate with the family. For example, it gives the clinician more opportunity to observe family interactions and individual behaviors or feelings. It permits the PCP to demonstrate active and empathetic listening.

- It allows the clinician to emphasize and to communicate important points to the family as he or she jots something down (eg, *"That's important,"* or *"I agree with you."*).

- It also permits the clinician to give a compliment as he or she writes something down (eg, *"Now that is really impressive!"*).

- It lets the family better observe the clinician's reactions as it looks for support, understanding, and respect. To the family, excessive note taking may appear to be a way for the clinician to "hide" his or her own feelings, or it may make the clinician appear distant and uninterested.

- Brief note taking appears friendlier and less clinical. In family meetings, the family usually wants a warm, supportive relationship in which the clinician "joins" the family as part of the therapeutic process. Excessive note taking can prohibit the formation of this relationship. When the members see that everything they say or do is recorded, they often feel uneasy, hesitant, and/ or self-conscious. They may even feel that the session isn't "confidential."

HUMOR

A stressed family is often somber and intent on solving its "problem." This seriousness can make it lose perspective so that its concerns appear worse than they are. The family members may not have laughed together for a long time, or they may have lost their sense of humor. Clinicians, in their attempt to be professional, sometimes contribute to the problem by taking themselves and their positions too seriously. Humor is used most effectively when the clinician can make fun of himself or herself. When the clinician models this concept to the family, the family members learn not to take themselves so seriously all the time and to "lighten up" and feel better, even temporarily.

Laughter and humor can change the family's perspective of the problem (eg, members might laugh at their efforts to resolve a problem or for being so worried over *"such a little problem"*). Parents often say, *"It feels good to laugh; we haven't done that for a long time."* If the clinician is uncertain about whether to use humor, he or she should not use it because the use of humor must be natural and spontaneous. It should also fit the family's mood and the clinician's style. Examples of appropriate times to use humor are listed below.

- During the family meeting, members may joke or say humorous things that elicit laughter from the others. The clinician should note this and encourage it, as follows:

  Clinician: *It's good to see you laugh. Do you all laugh much at home? What kinds of things make you laugh? Who has the sense of humor?*

- Families might say things that the clinician can use to promote laughter, such as:

  Parent: *I was so mad, I told him he was grounded for a month.*

  Clinician: *A month? How could you stand having him in the house all that time?*

Humor serves other purposes. A family can use humor to avoid pain or because family members do not recognize the severity of a problem. Humor is also used in hurtful ways (eg, making fun of another or playing practical jokes). Sometimes, the family scapegoat is the target of jokes. When the clinician detects these situations, he or she should respond appropriately by gently confronting the family to help it adopt a different perspective and a more healthy response to the family member who is the target.

SELF-DISCLOSURE

The clinician might disclose past or current personal experiences selectively and with discretion to demonstrate empathy and understanding. The clinician must first decide that sharing an experience really is appropriate for the situation and is beneficial to the family and that it does not harm the clinician–family relationship. The advantage of self-disclosure is that it can establish a more personal and trusting relationship between the clinician and the family. For example, the family with a parent–adolescent conflict might stimulate the clinician to disclose his or her own similar experience, as the following situation illustrates.

Clinician: *I can understand your problem because I had a similar problem with my teenager a few years ago.*

Parents (thinking to themselves): *He's been through this himself. He knows the pain we are feeling. He can understand where we're coming from.*

In another situation, a child might have a particular problem, such as poor athletic skills. The clinician might share that she also experienced this problem and how she learned to develop other interests and skills that earned her satisfaction and praise.

On the other hand, the clinician's self-disclosure can be problematic. The family may perceive the disclosure as a weakness which, in turn, may alter its view of the physician as the expert or the leader. Also, if the clinician talks too much about his or her own past, he or she is taking time and attention away from the family. If the clinician has any question or doubt about self-disclosure, he or she should avoid it.

Chapter 14

Techniques for Dealing With Difficult Families

*C*linicians often encounter "difficult" families, which consequently cause them to feel worn down and discouraged. These families, which may be chaotic, distrustful, angry, or depressed, frustrate and challenge the clinician. In these situations, the clinician must exert strong leadership, provide more structure to the meeting, be patient, give the family extra support, confront with empathy if necessary, and be sensitive to the idea that the family may have a hidden agenda that has yet to emerge. The clinician may also consider a referral or transferring a family's care to a trusted colleague.

Types of difficult families are listed in Box 14.1 and described in detail on the following page.

Box 14.1. Types of Difficult Families

- Chaotic family
- Discouraged family
- Family with a parent who "refuses" to attend the meeting
- Family that has difficulty adhering to the time limits of the visit
- Family with a hostile, angry parent
- Family member who lies
- Family with a confused member
- Family with a resistant family member
- Family that is reluctant to change
- Family that is stuck on problems or has unrealistic goals

CHAOTIC FAMILY

Some families are chaotic. They can be loud, overactive, and disorganized. They interrupt, talk over others, and have difficulty complying with requests and tasks in the meeting. These families can be good-natured, irritable, confused, or worried. The clinician establishes control by structuring the meeting and by setting rules early in the meeting to make it orderly. A few suggestions to accomplish this are listed below.

- Before the meeting begins, the clinician states a few rules.

   Clinician: *I'd like to explain a few rules that will make the session more comfortable and productive for you.*
   — Please let each person speak without interruption.
   — Only one person may speak at a time.
   — Please don't interrupt or talk over someone.
   — Speak for yourself, not for someone else.
   — Speak to the person you wish to communicate with instead of to me.

- Structuring also makes the session feel safe. Every member needs reassurance that the family meeting is a safe place to express thoughts and feelings without fear of blame, threats, punishment, criticism, or loss of the family's love and approval. The clinician introduces this below.

   Clinician: *The family meeting is a safe place where everyone can speak honestly without fear of being criticized. No one will be blamed or punished. Everyone's thoughts and feelings are important.*

   If one member yells, calls another member names, or accuses another, the clinician must quickly and firmly intervene.

   Clinician: *I know you feel very strongly about this, but I must ask you not to yell or call anyone names. Please tell us what you think or feel in a calm voice. You can do this without blaming anyone.*

- The clinician must help the family members cooperate by remaining neutral and not taking sides. Active listening and allowing each member approximately equal time to communicate conveys interest and neutrality. Sometimes, however, the clinician needs to be more direct.

   Clinician: *I want to say that I am not taking sides in this meeting. My role is to help you all work together and to provide any help in order for you to achieve your goal.*

- The clinician can structure the meeting if he or she keeps the family on its stated topic or points out its difficulty staying focused, as in the following situation:

   Clinician: *Let's go back to the topic that you agreed on as the one you wanted to discuss. We can talk about the other issue you raised at another* *time.* or *Can you see how the family jumps around from topic to topic? It appears that it is hard to stay on one topic.* or *Everyone seems to have a different agenda. Maybe this is one of the problems.*

- If the children run around and act disruptively, the clinician should let the parents respond first. If they do not respond or if they respond ineffectively, the clinician should ask them what they would like to do. Sometimes parents hesitate to respond firmly or angrily in the office, or they are waiting for "permission" from the clinician.

Clinician: *Is this what happens at home? What would you like to do when Johnny runs around and interrupts?*

- — The clinician can distract and calm children by offering them toys, books, or drawing materials to use in the room or in the hallway just outside the room.
- — Older children can play in the office playroom if one is available.
- — The clinician can determine if the child is hungry or if he or she needs a diaper change or to use the bathroom.
- — Some children calm down when sitting on their parents' laps or when addressed with a firm word.
- — The clinician should remind parents to bring snacks, toys, and books as necessary.
- — Sometimes leaving infants and children at home, if they are not actively involved in the meeting, works best.

DISCOURAGED FAMILY

Families seek help when they have experienced failure and disappointment, so they feel discouraged and hopeless. The interpersonal relationships have often been strained, and they have negative perceptions of others and themselves. When working with a discouraged family, the clinician should always acknowledge its feelings. A short discussion and/or ventilation of feelings often proves helpful. Then the clinician can initiate a search for individual and family strengths; the search for positives improves the family's perceptions by reminding it of its individual and family strengths and successes. This realization reduces the sense of hopelessness and the intensity of the negative feelings by shifting the focus from problems to solutions. The family's thoughts now might be that *"Yes, we may have some problems, but we also have strengths. We are doing something right."*

- The clinician helps the family find its strengths by making a "request." The request is an indirect compliment to the family because it implies that the clinician believes the family has past successes and forgotten strengths.

The requests may be about the following:

— About themselves. For example, the clinician may say, *"Julie, tell us something about yourself that you are proud of, that you recently did, or that makes you feel good."*

— About one member's perceptions of another. The clinician may ask a parent something such as, *"Ms Cohen, tell us something about Julie that you are proud of or that makes you happy."*

— About relationships. The clinician searches by saying, *"Julie, tell us about something enjoyable that you and your mom do together or did recently."* or *"Ms Cohen, tell us about some activity, errand, or chore that you and Julie have recently done together."*

• The solution-oriented questions. The clinician begins the interview with selected questions that emphasize strengths, possibilities, and solutions. Problem-oriented questions, which can perpetuate discouragement, should be asked later in the interview. The 3 solution-oriented questions described below include goal, exception, and scaling questions. The clinician should choose the one that best seems to fit the family. See Chapter 24.

— Goal questions. In exploring goals the clinician says, *"Let me begin with a different kind of question. If you could wish to make things better, what would you wish for?"* or *"What would you like to see happen by coming to this meeting?"* The clinician might use the magic wand with the child to facilitate these questions. See Chapter 28.

— Exception questions. To introduce these questions, the clinician begins by saying, *"Let's begin with a new kind of question. Suppose things were better, what would be different?"* or *"Tell me about a time when things were better, when the problem wasn't happening as much."*

— Scaling questions. The clinician uses the following process to ask these questions. He or she says, *"I'm going to begin our meeting with a different kind of question. On a scale of 1 to 10, 1 represents the worst things have been and 10 is the best things could be. Where are you right now?"* The clinician always uses the answer to initiate a search for strengths. *"So you are at 4. That's pretty good. Almost halfway there. You must be doing something right. Tell me what you are doing to be there."*

Everyone should participate so that a sense of cooperation, competence, and support is built.

FAMILY WITH A PARENT WHO "REFUSES" TO ATTEND THE MEETING

Clinicians often encounter families in which one parent refuses to attend the family meeting. The parent who is present at the meeting (or on the phone) speaks for the absent parent, reporting that the absent parent "refuses" to attend.

The clinician should consider the following possibilities and responses:

- The parent present in the meeting (or on the phone) may be deliberately excluding the other parent for many reasons, including possibly because they disagree about parenting, because the parents are experiencing marital conflict, or because the absent parent has a personal problem (eg, alcoholism, depression). The parent in the meeting may offer excuses, such as, *"He's not really involved"* or *"Her work schedule is too demanding."*

- This situation often represents the parents' inability to cooperate at home and thus represents part of the problem (eg, *"We can't agree on how to raise our child."*). The clinician should share his or her concern in one of the following ways: *"I sense that you might not want your spouse to attend the meeting."* or *"I sense that the inability for both of you to be here and work together is another form of your disagreement. I need you both to attend the meeting if I am to help you."*

- The absent parent deliberately chooses to not attend the meeting because he or she feels or thinks one of the following things:
  — He or she doesn't understand the purpose of the family meeting.
  — He or she doesn't think a family meeting is necessary.
  — The individual has had a "bad" experience in the past with mental health professionals.
  — The parent thinks a family meeting is "family therapy," which he or she doesn't want.
  — He or she feels that his or her authority is being challenged.
  — He or she worries about being blamed.

The clinician should ask the parent who is present about these issues and should suggest that the meeting be postponed until both parents agree to attend. He or she should explain the purpose of the family meeting and should emphasize the importance of participation from both parents.

If the absent parent still refuses to attend, the clinician should schedule a partial family meeting with the other members. Although this solution is not ideal, it may exert a positive influence on the whole family, like the "ripple effect" of a pebble dropped into a pond. Eventually, the absent parent may attend another meeting. This is preferable to the option of abandoning the family altogether or to making a referral that it is unlikely to accept. When a family gives up, the clinician should review the past meetings and find strengths in the family, even the fact that family members have attended the meetings. The clinician must be honest and ask the family for feedback, specifically has he or she done something "wrong," missed something, or made the family feel uncomfortable. The clinician must question whether any family member is trying to sabotage the meetings.

FAMILY THAT HAS DIFFICULTY ADHERING TO THE TIME LIMITS OF THE VISIT

Family meetings often do not proceed as efficiently or as predictably as routine medical visits. The clinician may be responsible for this (see Chapter 15). However, more often family members simply need time to "warm up"; once they do, they want to talk quite a bit.

The clinician should take the following steps:

- Remind the family early in the visit of the time limits of the visit and that other appointments will be scheduled for it. This takes pressure off the clinician (to complete the entire interview now) and the family (to offer all the explanations now) and creates an appropriate expectation for each visit.

  Clinician: *We have 30 minutes* (or *We have until 2:30*). *Let's spend this visit talking about your concerns. In the next visit, we'll talk about suggestions about what to do. We will schedule more visits after that.*

- Keep the focus on the purpose of this particular visit (eg, to discuss the problem and the goal that the family defined in the first part of the meeting). The clinician might say, *"Let's stick with the curfew problem and your goal of negotiating a compromise. We can talk about your other concerns at another meeting."*

- Place 2 clocks in the office; one should be easily visible to the family and the other to the clinician. This allows all participants to watch the time and to pace the visit and reduces the likelihood of the meeting ending abruptly, which is dissatisfying to everyone. Close to the end of the visit, the clinician should glance at or point to the clock and say, *"As you can see, it's almost time to end. I'd like to take the last few minutes to summarize our visit and answer your questions."* The readily visible clocks eliminate the need for the clinician to make furtive glances at a wristwatch, which can convey a sense of disinterest and haste.

- Signal the end by deliberately placing notes on the desk, shifting position, and stating, *"It's been a good meeting. Let's begin to wrap it up at this point."*

- Stand up if the family does not respond to these signals to end the meeting, and announce, *"I am sorry, but we need to conclude the meeting."*

- Arrange for the nurse to knock on the door or for the receptionist to call on the phone at a designated time to announce that the next patient is waiting.

- Refuse to explore new topics or to answer questions about new topics (eg, the family history or medications) at the end of a visit. These areas can be addressed at the next meeting.

FAMILY WITH AN ANGRY, HOSTILE PARENT

Sometimes in the office or clinic, a parent will yell or swear at the child and/ or yank, hit, or slap the child. A parent who acts angrily and aggressively with the child in the clinic may actually be signaling for help. The behavior is usually symptomatic of several issues: a situational, acute stress; inadequate parenting skills; or a chronic personal or family social–emotional problem. The clinician should never ignore this behavior. Instead, the clinician can do the following.

Hostility may be directed toward another family member, another person not present in the meeting, or at the clinician. Hostility is easy to recognize: words, tone, body language, facial expression. The clinician must deal with it immediately by acknowledging the member's feelings (eg, *"I sense that you are feeling uncomfortable in this meeting. Many family members feel this way initially in family meetings. Would you like to talk about this for a few minutes?"*). If the clinician does not deal with it immediately, he or she might "lose the interview."

- The clinician must recognize various causes of hostility, such as
  — Fear of diagnosis or illness.
  — Displaced hostility: The targeted person is an innocent target of negative transference (eg, patient is angry at pediatric care professional [PCP], prior experience with other professionals, school, parent, and sibling).
  — Fear of unwanted intimacy, own feelings, feelings toward another— wants to keep a distance.
  — Fear of dependence: The member wants to keep a distance from those who seem to have power, or the member has a fear of feeling inferior or failing; hostility and resentment often are generalized: don't ignore.
  — Habitual hostility and aggression as a coping style, or a way to maintain control.
  — Iatrogenic (problem caused by the PCP): The PCP appears to not be empathetic, involved, interested, or nonjudgmental, or appears to be taking sides.
  — If the child is hostile, it may be that he or she is brought under protest and feels he or she is the family scapegoat.
  — The PCP should be aware of transference and counter-transference and how that may affect a family member.

Suggestions to diffuse a family member's hostility or anger include

- The PCP could suggest that they take a break but not end the interview. For example, the clinician could say: *"It seems like things are uncomfortable now. Let's take a short break and resume the meeting in ten minutes."*
- Always Acknowledge Affect (AAA). The clinician might say, *"It is very challenging being a mother sometimes."* or *"It looks like you've had a hard day."*
- Briefly explore the immediate context of the behavior. For example, was the parent waiting a long time in the waiting room or examination room? Is the clinician running late? Did the parent have a difficult time at the registration desk? Is the child being especially difficult? Is the child hun-

gry and tired? Was the parent treated rudely by the receptionist, nurse, or clinician and therefore is taking his or her anger out on the child? If something occurred in the clinic, the clinician should apologize and should try to fix it later. For example, the clinician could say: *"I'm sorry for the delay. I know it is irritating, I realize you have been very patient and have a good reason to feel upset."*

- Ask if this (angry) behavior happens at home and, if so, how often. The clinician can ask, *"Does this happen at home or just when you are here?"* or *"How often does this happen at home?"*

- Ask if other stresses exist at home or work. The clinician can say, *"Are there things going on at home or at work that are stressful?"*

- Explore other ways for the parent to respond to the child. The clinician can respond with, *"I know it is difficult being in this small room with Johnny. Let me see if I can help out when he's demanding."*

- Explore a parenting technique for a similar situation at home. The clinician can do this by saying, *"When this happens at home, are there times that you respond calmly and more effectively?"*

- Remain nonjudgmental and supportive. The parent is very stressed, so the clinician should not lecture, moralize, embarrass, or challenge the parent. The clinician might say, *"I know this is a difficult situation, and I'll do all I can to make this day a successful meeting."*

- Ask about how the other parent or partner disciplines the child. For example, the clinician might say, *"How does your husband (wife, partner) handle things or respond to Johnny?"*

- Ask if the parent has a support system. The clinician can explore this with, *"When things are tough or you feel overwhelmed, do you have someone you can call for help and support? Who is this person?"*

- Intervene in a positive, yet authoritative manner. The parent needs guidance. The clinician can calmly take the child, sit the child on his or her lap, and engage the child in play. If possible, the clinician could let the child go to the playroom while the parent calms down. Not only does this response give the parent a break and a chance to talk to the clinician alone, but it also demonstrates or models a positive parenting technique. In effect, the clinician is saying, *"Kids can be frustrating sometimes. Let me show you another way to deal with this behavior."*

- The parent's angry behavior is often a call for help and provides an opportunity to offer more ongoing assessment and intervention. The clinician's response communicates empathy by saying, *"It's hard to be patient with a young child. It takes an extra effort and that's not easy. Let's schedule a meeting to help make things easier."*

FAMILY MEMBER WHO LIES

- Possible causes include fear, anger, shame, guilt, worry, lies for social gain, psychiatric illness, long history of lying (maybe to avoid abuse or punishment); despite history of difficulties and stress patient denies or minimizes problems. The clinician could say, *"For these meetings to be successful, we have to be frank and honest. Everything in this meeting is confidential."*
- Delicate situation: Suspect if history is internally inconsistent with probable facts or course of events or if family member contests answers. The clinician might say, *"This seems like a sensitive topic. I feel I'm getting mixed messages. The facts seem inconsistent and I am confused."*
- The PCP should inquire about behaviors that usually make one ashamed or guilty (eg, drugs, violence, or sex). The clinician could say, *"I know there are some delicate and personal issues involved, but we need to be honest with each other so these meetings meet your goals."*
- The PCP needs to get accurate information; be delicate; and avoid confrontation, judgment, and accusation. These will disrupt the relationship and lose the trust of the family. The clinician might tell the family, *"For us to work together, I need to get accurate and truthful information, and although this is somewhat difficult, it needs to be done."*
- The PCP should stage interventions. For example, the PCP should try not to confront in first interview. The PCP should not ignore the lie, but should seek the facts in the records and other activities. He or she should ask the patient to restate what the patient said, suggesting the clinician may have misunderstood or the family member misspoke. The clinician must try to resolve exaggeration or minimization of symptoms and facts. For example, the clinician could say, *"I know that we are discussing sensitive and personal issues. Oftentimes various family members do not know all the facts. I'd like us to try to clarify our thoughts and feelings, try not to exaggerate or cloud the truth."*

  If confrontation is needed, avoid accusatory or judgmental statements (eg, "Something puzzles me. You said you have no drinking problem but you were stopped for a DUI, or bottles were found in your room. Can you help me?")

Family With a Confused Member

- Possible causes include low cognitive ability, speech and language problems, memory problems, slow processing of information, disorganized thinking, too much contradictory input/information, depression, anxiety, and substance abuse. Emotions can fog facts and recall.
- The history may be scanty, partly true and unreliable, rambling, and incoherent, and the patient is over-talkative.

- The family member may feel frustrated, hostile, incompetent, and hesitant.
- The PCP should go slowly, stop and clarify in a short and simple manner, and re-explain the purpose of the meeting and the PCP role. The clinician should ask the family or a particular member if he or she understands and wants a repetition, or wants a clarification. Use short sentences and summarize often.
- The PCP should minimize psychological or medical jargon, and complicated words. He or she should choose words carefully, gather information in a logical sequential manner, interrupt the member at appropriate places, and help the member stay on topic (eg, *"Let's discuss this topic now and we can discuss others later."*) The clinician should not become tired, frustrated, lose concentration or rapport, and let the family member dominate the meeting even when done so unintentionally.
- The PCP should always try to maintain a positive affect, facial expressions, and tone of voice.

Family With a Resistant Member

- The clinician must ask if he or she has caused or provoked the resistance. He or she should ask the family member if sensitive or personal information is causing the resistance. The PCP should assure the family members that each has a right to his or her feelings and the clinician understands their confusion and resistance. The PCP should again remind the family that the meeting is confidential. This is normalizing resistance. For example, the clinician might say, *"In these family meetings it is necessary to explore sensitive and personal information. Is it possible that this is causing you to feel somewhat resistant or hesitant?"*
- The clinician, as a remedy, may switch from pursuing facts and information to sharing feelings. The clinician may need to sacrifice information for rapport to maintain the integrity of the interview. The clinician should minimize or ignore resistant behavior for the time being and use supportive language, voice, and body language to attempt to reduce the resistance. The clinician should note and share observations about the family's emotions and body language, *"It seems that some of you appear uncomfortable with this topic, and others seem more open to discussing it."*
- The clinician should assure the patient or the family member that any form of interaction would be helpful, and the clinician would welcome this in a nonjudgmental manner, *"I know this is difficult, but any kind of response from you would be very helpful and you won't be judged in any way."*

- The PCP should encourage the resistant family member and acknowledge every increment of progress, whether verbal or nonverbal. For example, the clinician might say, *"I appreciate that you are sharing a little bit."* or *"I notice that you seem more comfortable now."*
- The clinician should focus on what is important to the resistant family member now, and be flexible and ready to change topics or pace of the interview. The clinician should try to anticipate and avoid sources of resistance for now. The clinician should always monitor his or her own communication style, both verbal and nonverbal, and adapt the interview style to fit the family's style.
- The clinician should not argue with the family member.

FAMILY THAT IS RELUCTANT TO CHANGE

- Families that feel that the clinician is pushing them too fast are reluctant to change.
- Families also appear "reluctant" if the clinician does not observe their interactions, ignores "clues" and "messages" and, hence, misses opportunities to move the family forward and create change.
- Some families have compelling, powerful secrets and forces within the family system that prevent change (eg, families who maintain the symptom to preserve the family balance and to sustain their relationships).

When families are or appear reluctant, the clinician must consider these possible causes. If a family is maintaining the symptom, the clinician must decide whether to acknowledge or confront its need to maintain the symptom. If the PCP does not, he or she must then determine whether to change the topic for this meeting or discuss a smaller more realistic goal. The PCP can also decide whether to end the meeting and/or discuss a referral in a supportive manner.

FAMILY THAT IS STUCK ON PROBLEMS OR HAS UNREALISTIC GOALS

Sometimes families get stuck on problems or have unrealistic goals. A session or two may be needed to get them "unstuck." The family needs a new "map," which will create new directions and movement, to shift it off the problem and on to realistic goals. Table 14.1 offers a few suggestions for dealing with this type of family.

Table 14.1. Getting the Family Off the Problem and on to Realistic Goals

Family	Clinician
Perseverates on problem	Emphasizes and rephrases goals and exception questions
Discusses many problems; can't prioritize or agree	*Helps family focus* "What is the most important issue *now?*" *Guides family* "I think communicating better with each other is more important than taking out the garbage. What do you think?"
States vague goals ("to get along better")	*Helps family specify goal behaviors* "What would you each be doing when you two are getting along better?"
States grand, unrealistic goals ("to always be a happy family")	*Helps family construct realistic goals* "What would be the first hint that you were beginning to be a happy family? Let's work on that first."
Talks of negative behaviors as a goal (less of or the absence of a problem: "not to mess up in school")	*Asks exception questions to state goal as a positive behavior* "When you are not messing up in school, what are you doing instead? When did you last do well in school? What did you do differently? How would your teacher know?"
Relies on someone else changing ("If only my son would obey.")	*Elicits description of parent's own behavior in the relationship and how parent behavior influences the child* "So suppose your son was obeying, what would you be doing differently? How could your behavior help him obey?"

Chapter 15

Common Pitfalls to Avoid

*P*itfalls are "breakdowns" in the clinician's interviewing. These problems are naturally part of the learning process, so the clinician should consider them as opportunities for growth. If the clinician does not encounter occasional problems, he or she is missing something and is not monitoring the quality of the interview, as reflected in the family's behavior, his or her own behavior, and family–clinician interactions.

As a general rule, to monitor his or her behavior and be aware of pitfalls the clinician should always

- Ask the family for feedback about the meeting.
- After the meeting (post-interview phase), the clinician should evaluate how the meeting went and also note how his or her behavior influenced the outcome of the meeting.
- Measure the family's progress and use that to gauge his or her effectiveness. This can only be accomplished with follow-up visits.
- Seek advice or supervision from a colleague if a second opinion is needed.

Several common pitfalls are listed in Box 15.1.

Box 15.1. Pitfalls to Avoid

- Too much information
- Slow pace
- Fast pace
- Clinician judges and takes sides
- Clinician has a "rescue fantasy"
- Clinician becomes part of a dysfunctional system
- Clinician does not search for strengths
- Clinician does not protect his or her personal life

Common pitfalls and solutions are described below.

- **Too much information.** Families can give and/or clinicians can request too much information. For example, the family might recount numerous, detailed examples of the problem behavior when one or two examples sufficiently reveal the problem. Too much data overwhelm the clinician, distract the family, consume valuable time, exhaust everyone, and prevent deeper exploration of the family context. The clinician therefore must limit the content and must focus more on the process.

- **Slow pace.** The clinician paces the interview too slowly. For example, the pediatric care professional (PCP) is reluctant to explore the family context and assess family functioning so that the interview does not move beyond the friendly chatting of the first step (see Step 1: Engaging the Family, page 76). To remedy this, the clinician must actively monitor the pace and must proceed to the second step (see Step 2: Understanding the Family, Its Concern, and Its Goal, page 81) as soon as he or she has greeted the family, explained the purpose of the meeting, and started the "joining" process.

- **Fast pace.** At times, the clinician paces the interview too quickly and fails to begin with "join the family" (form a therapeutic alliance) and to explain the purpose of the meeting. As a result, the quality of the meeting diminishes. Rushing the interview (not scheduling enough time for interview sessions) can be perceived by the family as a lack of empathy, respect, and/or professionalism. The clinician should monitor and adjust the pace to fit the allotted time; schedule more time for the interview; and schedule more meetings, if necessary.

- **Clinician judges and takes sides.** The clinician can develop affinities or sympathies for a particular family member and can side with that member against another, a phenomenon that is not uncommon. For instance, a clinician can side with a parent(s) against a child or with a child against a parent(s). However, the clinician must maintain an impartial family systems perspective, so he or she should review his or her performance in the post-interview phase and should ask the family for feedback (*"Does everyone feel they were treated equally or given equal time?"* and *"Does anyone feel blamed or picked on?"*).

- **Clinician has a "rescue fantasy."** The clinician is moved and/or motivated by the family's problems and pain. The clinician promises to try to help the family more than he or she can or more than the family desires because the clinician feels compelled to "save" the family. Families become disappointed when the clinician can't keep promises to help them, so they may become "resistant" to further efforts or end the relationship. Disappointment and resistance from the family are signals to the clinician. When the clinician detects these signals, he or she needs to assess whether or not he or she is trying to meet some personal needs at the expense of the family. If this is the case, the professional relationship may have to end if the clinician cannot adjust.

- **Clinician becomes part of a dysfunctional system.** The clinician is drawn into acting as certain family members do in the conflict. The clinician develops the same feelings of helplessness or anger or the same behaviors that are part of the problem in the family system. The clinician may join in family arguments as if he or she were one of the members. As a result, the clinician ceases to be an effective force in the family system treatment plan. To avoid this pitfall, the clinician must constantly monitor his or her own behavior, tone of voice, use of language, and facial expression, and not give undue attention or time to a particular family member. Remaining "apart" and above the conflict is essential to remaining as an independent advocate for the family.

- **Clinician does not search for strengths.** At times, the clinician fails to explore the family's resources and the strengths it brings with it to the meeting (eg, past successes, supports, commitment, resilience, and love for one another). Families need to hear "good news" and to be reminded of their strengths because they have often forgotten or have discounted them. Families feel even more discouraged and unmotivated if the clinician dwells only on their problems.

- **Clinician does not protect his or her personal life.** In this scenario, the clinician encourages families to call at any time of the day or night, schedules appointments during non-clinic hours, and responds to every crisis. Because of this, the clinician becomes overwhelmed and consumed. Seeing too many families exceeds the clinician's "available" time, resources, and patience. When this happens, both the clinician and the family lose. Clinicians must "protect" themselves by specifying when they are available and how the family should contact them, and by limiting the number of families in their practice.

SECTION C SUMMARY

Working with families is not always smooth, easy, or successful for the clinician or the family. Sometimes the clinician will experience disappointment and failure. These setbacks are part of the learning process for the clinician. To be successful, the PCP should review the skills often and monitor his or her progress. This section described 4 categories of strategies with which to increase the chances of a successful interview: effective communication skills (eg, permitting silence); specific interviewing techniques to facilitate a successful interview (eg, remaining neutral), strategies for dealing with difficult families (eg, the chaotic family), and common pitfalls to avoid (eg, the clinician judges and takes sides).

Skills Checklist

Discuss

- Be aware of one's own interviewing style and self-monitor oneself in the interview and the post-interview phase.
- Review the techniques of successful family interviewing.
  — Communication skills
  — Specific interviewing techniques
  — Techniques for dealing with difficult families
  — Pitfalls to avoid
- Review your own family cases and think of the effective techniques you may have used.
- Consider how you might improve your family interviewing.
- Ask a peer or mentor to sit in with you or observe you with a family and then provide feedback.
- Offer to observe a peer or mentor.

The Family Interview: A Detailed Description

Chapter 16

The 4 Steps of a Family Interview With Case Studies

*T*he family interview is a semi-structured diagnostic and psychotherapeutic goal-oriented conversation between the clinician and the family. It also serves to encourage a conversation among family members. The interview generally follows a 4-step sequence: (1) engaging the family; (2) understanding the family, their concerns and goals; (3) working with the family; and (4) concluding the interview. Each step contains its own set of questions and specific elements.

This chapter uses a case study to illustrate and describe the 4 steps of the family interview and the various questions/elements of each step (Box 16.1). This guide will help the pediatric care professional (PCP) organize the interview so that it is productive, satisfying, and time-efficient.

Box 16.1. The 4 Steps of the Family Interview

1. Engaging the family (alliance formation)
2. Understanding the family, its concerns, and its goals
3. Working with the family (the therapeutic phase: direct interventions; helping the family focus on its goals and develop its own solutions)
4. Concluding the family meeting (summarizing, complimenting, planning the next meeting)

NO ONE WAY TO CONDUCT A FAMILY INTERVIEW

The interview is an individualized, dynamic, flexible process shaped by a variety of clinician and family factors. The steps and questions outlined in this chapter are a general guide. There is no standard interview approach.

Therefore, each PCP must develop his or her own interviewing style and individualize the interview to fit the family, PCP skills, and PCP time limitations. The PCP does not need to include all the aspects of each step, nor is it feasible to do so. The PCP can also shift back and forth from one step to another as the interview dictates.

Even though many questions are listed in this case study, asking all of them is often not necessary or feasible. The clinician should modify the content and sequence of the interview appropriately as conditions dictate. The clinician can select particular questions (or add new ones) for use in particular situations. He or she must also acknowledge that carrying out a complete, initial interview in one session may not be possible. The clinician may use 2 visits as follows: the first 2 steps (engaging the family and understanding the family) might be completed in the first visit, and the next 2 steps (working with the family and concluding the meeting) might be finished in the second visit. Follow-up visits are always needed.

Case Study 16.1: The Family With 2 Sons Experiencing Intense Sibling Rivalry

The father of 2 boys, Alex (9) and Rodney (11), called the clinician stating, *"My sons are always fighting. It's gotten so bad that I worry about them having a good relationship; it's really strained our home life. We don't know what to do."* The PCP knows the boys well but does not know the family well. The PCP feels this problem would be best resolved with a family meeting. He suggests this to the father, who agrees.

Step 1: Engaging the Family

The first step in the family interview is engaging the family. Engaging the family requires forging a trusting alliance with every member of the family—the PCP begins to "join" with the family as soon as they meet. Although the family already knows the PCP, this step is critical because the nature of the relationship between the PCP and the entire family strongly influences the outcome. The PCP is meeting other family members for the first time in a family context. This is different than the traditional child-centered encounter. In this step of the interview, the clinician should remember several interviewing strategies to establish the therapeutic alliance (Box 16.2).

**Box 16.2. Establishing the Alliance:
4 Key Aspects of Engaging the Family**

1. Partnership
2. Respect
3. Validation
4. Support

- Partnership means working together. From the beginning, the clinician works with the family in a problem-solving partnership, which he or she establishes by saying, *"How can I help you?"* or *"We'll work on this together."*
- Respect is conveyed by nonjudgmental acknowledgment and acceptance of the family's complaint, efforts, values, strengths, resilience, and other qualities. A compliment such as, *"I admire your commitment to your family."* or *"I respect your family values,"* communicates respect.
- Validation implies legitimizing the family's concerns, feelings, and actions. The clinician ensures that the family does not perceive itself or its problems as abnormal, unrealistic, or hysterical. He or she emphasizes this in responses to the family by making comments like, *"You have a right to feel as you do."* or *"Anyone would have done the same thing."*
- Support indicates ongoing help. The clinician needs to assure the family that he or she will work with it until things are better and that the family members can depend on his or her continuing support and advocacy. The clinician should let the family know this by making statements such as, *"I will help you as long as it takes."* or *"You can always call me whenever you need to."*

Engaging the family includes building the relationship and developing the therapeutic alliance between the family and the clinician. Relationship building, which is the first step, continues and develops throughout all subsequent interviews. It is an ongoing process.

The 5 elements of engaging the family are greeting, social conversation, identifying the family leader, explaining the purpose of the meeting, and estimating the number of visits (Box 16.3).

Box 16.3. Engaging the Family: Allow 3 to 5 Minutes for This Step[a]

- **The greeting:** Be warm and welcoming, address everyone by name, invite the family members to sit where they wish.
- **Social conversation:** Talk briefly to each member, make each feel involved and respected, join with the family.
- **Identifying the family leader:** Identify who is in charge.
- **Explaining the purpose of the meeting:** Appreciate the family context, use the family as a resource, explain to the family how this is different from the typical medical visit.
- **Estimating the number of visits:** Decide how many visits will be needed and how much time each visit will require. This relieves the pressure the family feels to get the problem solved in one visit.

[a]The 3- to 5-minute time allotment for this step of the visit is only an approximation.

The Greeting

The greeting, the first contact between the family and the clinician, should be warm and welcoming to help put the family at ease. Every member must be greeted by name and with a smile, eye contact, and physical contact. Children are called by their first names (not "your son," "he," or "she") and should be acknowledged with either a pat on the shoulder or a handshake. Parents and other adults should be greeted with formal names or titles and handshakes. At this point, the clinician also introduces himself or herself using the name or title with which he or she would prefer to be addressed.

If the clinician greets the family members in the waiting room and then escorts them to the room that is going to be used for the family meeting, he or she should start the social conversation at that point. He or she could say, *"It's good to see you,"* or *"Thank you for being so prompt."* He should not ask *"How are you doing?"* because that is part of the next step (understanding the family) and should be carried out at the appropriate step. The clinician should not hurry down the hall several paces in front of the family, silently leading them to the room while glancing through the chart. Taking a few minutes to review the chart before greeting the family or reviewing it with the family members in the office is preferable.

Once in the room where the chairs are arranged in a loose semi-circle, the family members should be invited to sit where they wish. A child may prefer to sit on a parent's lap. The seating arrangement itself may reveal something about family relationships (eg, the child who sits next to his father and far from his mother may be indicating his emotional closeness to the father and distance from the mother).

Case Study 16.1 (continued)

The clinician has followed the boys for several years so she felt she knows them. She doesn't feel that she knows the mother well, and she has never met the father in previous visits.

Social Conversation

In this element, the clinician talks with each family member, making a connection with each individual so that each one feels important, involved, and acknowledged. These few minutes of social conversation, which are especially useful in the first meeting when the family is the most nervous and hesitant, establish personal contact between the clinician and each member, help the clinician begin to know them, and relax the family. This time of informal "living room talk" permits the family members to settle down, to gather their thoughts, and to feel comfortable in the family session.

Starting with someone other than the "identified patient" (the member with "the problem") is best. Starting with members who are the least well-known to the clinician makes them feel involved early in the session. The clinician might preface his or her questions with the following statement, *"Before we start, I'd like to get to know you a little."*

Families often enter the room already engaged in conversation (eg, the traffic conditions it encountered driving to the office, daily activities, or plans following the visit). The clinician can often use those topics to begin the social conversation. For example, overhearing an ongoing conversation, he or she could say, *"I heard you talking about playing sports after school. What sport do you play?"*

Case Study 16.1 (continued)

Clinician (to the father): *I'm glad we have a chance to meet. I've enjoyed knowing your family.*

Identifying the Family Leader in the Hierarchy

The clinician must identify the family leader and make an alliance with him or her. The mother usually makes most of the child-rearing decisions and may also be the leader (the member who is ultimately "in charge" of the concern). However, the leader can also be the father, a parent's partner, or a grandparent who lives with or near the family. The alliance is crucial because this individual's support greatly influences the family's adaptability and cooperation. If the family leader is not yet known or is not present, he or she must be identified early in the interview.

Case Study 16.1 (continued)

Clinician (to the parents): *Mr Brown, you and I spoke on the phone about this appointment, but who generally makes decisions about the children?*
Father: *We both do.*
Mother: *I do more of the day-to-day things, but we are both concerned about this issue and agree on seeking help.*

Explaining the Purpose of the Meeting

Explaining that the purpose of the meeting is to understand the family context in which the problem arises helps the family realize how this meeting differs from a typical medical visit. The clinician must clearly explain that the discussion will not focus only on the child and "the problem." The members must understand that everyone's input is needed to yield a better understanding of the concern and the goal, and to provide better solutions. Sometimes children have not been told the purpose of the meeting, or they think it is "to make them behave." The clinician should correct these assumptions and should assure them that the focus is not on the symptoms or to blame any one family member. The clinician should not proceed with the meeting until the family clearly understands its purpose and appears comfortable with the shift from the "identified patient" to the family context.

Families (understandably) are uncertain and nervous about the purpose of the family meeting. The clinician can explain the purpose in the following way, *"I'd like to explain the purpose of the family meeting. All families face problems from time to time and need help solving them. We're having this meeting so that everyone can understand the issue, agree on a goal, and work together to make things better. As a family you have many strengths you can use to help resolve this issue. We're not here to blame anyone. This meeting has two parts. In the first part, everyone will talk about the concern that brings the family here and let's see if you all agree. Then we'll talk about your goal and how to achieve it, or at least start to make things better. Everyone needs to participate. If you don't want to talk at first that is okay, but after awhile I do want to hear from everyone."*

Case Study 16.1 (continued)

Clinician: *Does everyone know why we are meeting?*

Rodney: *Because I have a problem, and they want you to fix me.*

Clinician (to Rodney): *I want to remind you that you do not have "a problem." The whole family shares a concern and we're here to work on it together.*

Clinician (to the family): *Let me explain the purpose of this meeting.*

Estimating the Number of Visits

Most clinicians do not have enough time to conduct a complete initial interview in one visit. Early in the first visit, the clinician should estimate the number of visits that will be necessary and then should tell the family. This approximation might be based on prior knowledge of the family, on the parent's phone call, or on the nature of the presenting concern from the early discussion in the first meeting. Informing the family that sufficient time exists to discuss the concern and possibly their goal (eg, one or two visits for the complete initial interview and then a number of follow-up visits) is very reassuring to them. This removes considerable pressure and strain from both the family and the clinician. On the other hand, the PCP can "condense" the initial interview and later he or she might "go back" and seek other information.

Duration of Visits

Generally, an initial interview requires 40 to 60 minutes depending on the (apparent) complexity of the problem. The clinician can schedule this interview as 1 visit or as 2 visits of 20 to 30 minutes each. The number of follow-up visits varies. Each requires 20 to 30 minutes.

Case Study 16.1 (continued)

Clinician: *We'll need two visits to start off with and then schedule a few shorter visits afterward.*

Step 2: Understanding the Family, Its Concern, and Its Goal

The centerpiece of this step is understanding both the family and its concern. This step of the family meeting contains 2 parts: exploring the family structure and function and exploring the family's problem or concern within the family context. Helping the family to define its goals is also a key aspect of Step 2 (Box 16.4). The definition of the goal might need to be repeated, clarified, and redefined in subsequent meetings. (See Chapter 24.)

Box 16.4. Understanding the Family: Allow 20 to 30 Minutes for This Step[a]
- Exploring the family structure and function
- Exploring the family's concern and goal

[a]These time limits are only an approximation.

Exploring the Family Structure and Function

To explore the family structure and function, the clinician must observe the family's interactions and ask about the family composition, activities they share, the structure (eg, the hierarchy, roles, and coalitions), communication patterns, and family perceptions of the concern and of each other (Box 16.5).

Box 16.5. Exploring the Family Structure and Function
- Observe the family's pattern of interactions.
  - Content
  - Process
- Ask about the family.

Observing the family. The clinician's observations should begin when he or she greets the family and should continue throughout the visit(s). Observations also include information and impressions provided by the parent's initial phone call. The clinician should note both the content and the process of the family's interactions and communication. *Content* is defined as the verbal message, or the "what," of the communication. *Process* is the way in which the content is delivered—both the verbal and nonverbal message—

or the "how" of the communication and interaction. The clinician should observe the family with the following questions in mind:

- *What is the leader's style?*
  — How does he or she assert leadership (authoritarian, authoritative, loud, quiet, permissive)?
  — Is this person the most appropriate leader in this situation?
  — How does this person accept alternative suggestions, disagreement, praise, cooperation, and lack of cooperation?
  — Does the family respect the leader?
- *What is the family hierarchy?* Hierarchy can be established by the following information:
  — Who attends the meeting? Who makes decisions?
  — How do the other family members react to the leader?
  — Are "power," decision-making, and leadership shared appropriately?
  — What "role" does each member play in the "problem" and the resolution?
  — Does sharing change the hierarchy or family subsystems?
  — Do power struggles for leadership occur?
- *What do the family's nonverbal communications reveal?* The clinician should closely observe the following behaviors and interactions:
  — How do the family members enter the room and greet the clinician?
  — What is the seating arrangement? Who is sitting next to whom?
  — Are the parents sitting together or apart?
  — How is each member dressed? What is the general appearance?
  — What do facial expressions, eye contact, body postures communicate?
  — Do the members touch one another?
  — Are the family members relaxed or tense?
  — Do the members drift off, sit still, pay attention, or become fidgety?
  — How does the family send nonverbal messages to each other?
  — How do they respond to each other and to the clinician (eg, behaviors, moods, facial expressions)?
  — How does the family conclude the meeting and "say" goodbye?
- *What do the family's verbal communications reveal?* The clinician should note the following aspects:
  — Who initiates the communications?
  — How are the communications received by other family members?
  — What happens immediately after the communication? What does each family member say or not say?
  — Do members need "permission" to communicate certain topics?
  — What types of communication are cut off?
  — Who cuts off the communication?
  — How do family members both listen and speak to the clinician?
  — Do they all volunteer to talk?

— Do they listen to one another?

— Do they listen with empathy?

— Do they acknowledge each other's feelings?

— Do they talk to each other or only to the clinician?

— How do they handle interruptions and disruptions?

— What is not said in the meeting?

- *How does the family carry out discussions and tasks in the meeting?* (Tasks can include discussing a problem, sharing feelings, negotiating a goal, planning an activity, or [re]assigning roles.)

  — Does everyone participate, or does one person do everything?

  — Can the family create a plan for doing the task?

  — How are rules for doing the task formed and communicated?

  — Who participates in forming the plan?

  — Does sharing power and responsibility cause a breakdown in completing the task?

  — How does the family react to suggestions?

  — How age-appropriate and constructive are "duties" or work assignments?

  — Who assigns them and how?

  — Is the performance of the task basically leaderless?

- *What "roles" does each family member play during a discussion task and at home?*

  — By what process were they assigned or assumed?

  — Do these roles remain set, or do they change?

  — Does anyone sabotage the task? If so, who?

  — Who provides minimal support for the task?

  — Who does most of the work?

- *How does the family adapt during a discussion of the task?*

  — How does the leader of the task adapt to new task requirements and changes in the participants' behavior?

  — Is the family flexible?

  — Can family members correctly determine that the discussion or task should end for one or more of the following reasons?

    ▪ Someone is not feeling good.

    ▪ They cannot perform an assigned "job."

    ▪ Time is running out.

  — How does the family (and each member in it) react when a task cannot be completed?

  — How does the family treat the one who does not do his or her part?

  — Were harmful coalitions formed (did 2 or more members side against other family members)?

  — Does one (or more) family member(s) appropriately or inappropriately "rescue" another family member while doing the task?

- *What are the family's emotions during the discussion or task?*
  - — Does the family experience joy or accomplishment?
  - — Do the members express or demonstrate joy, approval, affection, anger, and/or sadness?
  - — How do they express these feelings?"
  - — How do they respond to one another's feelings?

Case Study 16.1 (continued)

The clinician notes that the parents sit together and that Alex is sitting close to his mother. Rodney, however, moved his chair to be as far as possible from the rest of the family. The family mood is serious, and the boys seem hesitant to talk. The father sighs as he sits down and says, *"I feel relieved that we are finally sitting down together to deal with this."* The mother initiates most of the conversation and appears to be the leader.

Asking about the family. In addition to observing the family's interactions, the clinician learns more about the family structure and function with the judicious use of just a few questions. Comprehensive fact-gathering questioning is neither necessary nor advisable, as the family usually divulges information in the course of the meeting without needing to be asked. Examples of questions that can be asked include the following:

- Who lives at home?
- Who is in charge at home?
- How do the siblings get along?
- How is the marriage/partnership?
- Is the marriage/partnership affected by the concern?
- Is the concern affected by the marriage/partnership?
- Who else cares for the children?
- Who are the extended family members?
- Where do extended family members live, and what is their relationship with the family?
- What does the family do together? Evenings? Vacations? For fun?
- Do they have any traditions? Holidays? Church or temple?
- Are there any social and environmental (outside) stresses on the family system?

Case Study 16.1 (continued)

Clinician: *Does anyone else live at home?*

Mother: *Just us. But all of the boys' grandparents live close by.*

Clinician: *Are they supportive? Do they help out?*

Father: *Very. My father always offers advice.*

Clinician (seeking clarification): *What kind of advice?*

Father: *How to raise the kids.*

The clinician makes a mental note to follow up on this comment because it seems related to the stated problem. But she has noted the family's mood and wants to acknowledge and understand it.

Clinician (exploring the mood): *I notice that everyone seems very serious.*

Mother: *Home life is tense.*

Clinician (acknowledging the tension): *Yes, I can see that. This must be a very difficult time for the family.*

Father: *It is. This fighting is not what we want as a family.*

Clinician (emphasizing the family context and being supportive): *That's why we're meeting as a family. We want to understand the issues better. It's apparent that everyone is affected. And as a family, you have the resources to resolve this concern.*

Exploring the Family's Concern and Goal

The 4 components of exploring the family's concern are (1) describing the concern and agreeing on it, (2) describing a goal and agreeing on it, (3) exploring past attempts/advice to resolve the concern, and (4) keeping the family focused on the goal (Box 16.6).

The clinician should have already discussed the purpose of the meeting. Now family members should state their own perceptions of the concern and should set a goal for the family, briefly describing the concern and agreeing on it with the aid of the clinician's leadership and experience.

Box 16.6. Exploring the Concern and the Goal

- Describing the concern and agreeing on it
- Describing the goal and agreeing on it
- Identifying family patterns that maintain the concern
- Exploring past attempts/advice to resolve the concern
- Keeping the family focused on the goal

Case Study 16.1 (continued)

Clinician: *First I'd like each of you to briefly describe the issue in just a few words. We'll discuss it in more detail in a few minutes. Who would like to begin?*

The clinician deliberately does not want to ask the boys first because she does not want to focus initially on the "identified patients."

Both parents: *The kids are always fighting.*

Clinician (inviting one of the boys to get involved): *What do you think, Alex?*

Alex: *I don't like fighting, but I have to.*

Clinician (clarifying): *You "have to"?*

Alex: *He picks on me. He starts it.*

Rodney: *We're just playing, but it's not my fault.*

Clinician: *Rodney, what do you think the concern is?*

Rodney: *The fighting and the lousy feelings.*

Father: *Maybe it's just a boy thing. I fought with my brother when I was young. But they fight too much.*

Clinician (attempting to be sure they agree about the "problem" and the goal): *Although you all seem to have different views, do you all feel that "fighting" is a concern and that "home life is tense"* (using the mother's phrase)?

The family agrees that these are the problems.

The clinician should now ask them about their goal. Describing and negotiating a goal serves 2 purposes. (See Chapter 24.)

- The goal helps the family members share with one another the behavior they want or need. The clinician might say, *"What would you like to achieve with these meetings?"*
- Reminding the family of its goal helps the clinician redirect the interview if and when the interview reverts to being problem-focused or too acrimonious, divisive, and accusatory. For example, the clinician might get the meeting back on track by saying, *"Remember that your goal is to have the boys play together. Let's go back to discussing how that can happen."* Some families become so fixated on the problem that they do not think about a goal. In those cases, the clinician needs to make an extra effort to help the family focus on its goal.

Case Study 16.1 (continued)

Clinician: *Now that you've stated your concern, I'd like to ask about your goal. What would you like to happen in your family?*

The family was silent. The clinician waited about 15 seconds.

Father: *What do you mean?*

Clinician: *If "home life" weren't so tense, what would be happening instead?*

Mother: *The kids would not be fighting.*

Clinician (helping the family restate the goal as a desirable behavior): *What would you see if they were not fighting?*

Father: *There would be peace in the house.*

Clinician (helping each family member specify his or her role in achieving the goal): *What would each of you be doing if there was peace in the house?*

Father: *We'd be doing chores and activities together. We'd feel comfortable.*

Alex: *I want Rodney to stop beating me up.*

Rodney: *I wouldn't be blamed for the fighting.*

Clinician (to help the mother, Alex, and Rodney state their goals in positive terms): *Could you tell us all what you want instead of fighting, instead of being beat up, and instead of being blamed?*

Mother: *I'd like the boys to play together after school.*

Alex: *I wish Rodney would play with me and not beat me up.*

Rodney: *I want Dad to know it's not my fault.*

Clinician (attempting to be sure they agree on a goal): *It sounds like you all want the same things: the boys playing together, feeling comfortable, and no one being blamed. Is that right?*

Rodney: *I want to play with Alex, not fight with him.*

Clinician (emphasizing the family meeting purpose): *That's one reason you're all here.*

The members look at each other silently.

Father (asking the family): *Is that right?*

The mother, Rodney, and Alex all nod.

In this exchange, the clinician helps the family focus on one goal. Since the boys' fighting appears to be the central problem, the logical goal is having the boys play together. After a brief conversation, the family agrees that this is their current goal.

Once the goal has been agreed on, the clinician should help the family focus on more goal description than talk of the concern. It is very common for families to fall back into "problem talk," and the clinician must constantly remind them to focus on the goal.

Family members often talk to the clinician about another's behaviors. They "report" their perceptions and feelings to the clinician. A major goal of the meeting is to get the members to communicate with each other. The clinician must remind them to look at and talk to each other. *"I'd like you to look at Rodney and tell him what you'd like to see happen."*

Case Study 16.1 (continued)

Clinician (seeking clarification): *What exactly do you all mean by "fighting"?*

The family explains that fighting means name calling and pushing. These activities have been going on for about a month; they used to occur only once or twice a week, but now they are happening almost daily. Most occurrences are after school during the few hours that the boys are home alone, so the parents are not sure who starts things. Lately the disagreements have intensi-fied to occasional punching; Alex often comes to his parents in tears.

Father (speaking to the clinician): *I've really had it. This is not what I want family life to be like.*

Clinician: *I'd like to ask all of you to address each other, not me. Could you look at your family and tell them that?*

The father does so. They are quiet.

The father's expression of his feelings is important. He has expressed both his frustration and his disappointment. The family "heard" him.

Mother: *I am sure we can do something, but I must admit that I'm lost. For a while I spanked Rodney, but I felt badly afterward so I stopped.*

Clinician (exploring this spontaneous disclosure of behavior and feelings): *Does Rodney know that?*

Mother: *This is the first time I've said this.*

Clinician (encouraging family communication): *Could you tell him now?*

Mother: *Rodney, I am sorry for the spanking. I feel badly for both of us.*

Rodney's eyes well up with tears. The mother reaches out and takes his hand. The clinician and family are silent.

This interaction was significant. The mother and son shared feelings verbally (mother) and nonverbally (Rodney).

Families often repeat behaviors that maintain the problem. As they work harder, louder, and longer, they become tired, impatient, and frustrated. These patterns of interaction are often passed from one generation to another. To help the family change these entrenched patterns, the clinician should identify them and share his or her observations with the family.

Case Study 16.1 (continued)

Clinician: *What do you do when the fighting occurs?*

The parents describe their patterns of behavior. When a fight has occurred, Alex usually comes to the mother; she, feeling that this is a father–son issue, asks her husband to "do something." The father, remembering how his father had raised him, tells Alex to "be tough and fight back."

However, recently when Alex came to him in tears, the father began to feel that Rodney was being too rough, so he has begun to scold him.

Mother: *I know spanking doesn't help. My parents spanked me, and I hated it.*

Rodney: *You yell at me too!*

The clinician made a mental note of the fact that, although the spanking had ceased, the yelling continues and that it is both a symptom and a cause of family stress.

Clinician (using an insight-oriented question): *Do you see a connection between how you were raised and your own parenting practices?*

The mother states that she does now that it has been pointed out.

Clinician (to the mother): *Does your behavior change anything?*

Mother: *It only makes the situation even more unhappy.*

Clinician (to the boys): *Let's hear from you.*

The boys start to argue and blame each other for the fighting. To help them refocus, the clinician reminds them of the stated goal to work together and not blame or hurt each other. Alex says that he felt that he was being picked on, so he usually told his father that Rodney was starting the fights.

Rodney says that he felt that he was unfairly blamed. He resented the spanking and the scolding and would tell Alex afterward, *"I'm going to get you for tattling to Dad."*

The clinician encourages a dialogue between Rodney and his father about Rodney's feelings. Then she acknowledges Rodney's feelings toward Alex and emphasizes again the purpose of the meeting, which is not to hurt or blame but to work together to achieve their goal.

Clinician (exploring the father's parenting history to understand the family context and the father's behaviors better): *Could you tell me more about how your parents raised you?*

Father: *My father always told us to settle our differences ourselves, even if it meant fighting. He wanted us to be "tough" and not "sissies."*

Exploring past attempts/advice to resolve the concern. This line of inquiry seeks to determine what, if any, attempts or advice the family has used in the past and helps to further define the goal. The answers inform the clinician about the appropriateness of the attempts/advice, each member's efforts, and the outcomes. Did each member cooperate and follow the advice or did one or more members disagree with it?

Case Study 16.1 (continued)

Clinician: *What else have you tried in the past?*

The parents state that they had punished Rodney by taking away TV time because he seems to be "starting the fights," but that it didn't help.

Rodney appears to be the scapegoat, the one who is usually blamed and, consequently, the clinician thinks he might have a negative self-image.

Clinician: *Have you spoken with Rodney's and Alex's teachers or sought professional help?*

The family has not sought any outside help.

Clinician (following up on the father's statement that he followed his father's advice; she is trying to find out if this maintained or eased the problem): *Has anyone offered advice?*

Father: *My father gives us advice. We don't really ask him, but we go along with it when he offers it.*

The paternal grandfather had strongly advised the father to "let the boys fight it out." He wanted grandsons who could "handle things like strong men do."

Clinician: *How does the advice change the problem?*

The father laughs uncomfortably and shrugs his shoulders.

Mother: *They fought even harder and hurt each other. That's what's happened.*

Clinician: *Has anything helped?*

Mother (sounding very discouraged): *Nothing I can think of.*

Clinician: *Were there any changes in the family about the time the fighting started or intensified? Any recent stresses like health or job problems or marital tensions?*

The family denies any changes.

Clinician (to Alex and then Rodney): *Have you had any difficulties at school or with friends?*

Alex denies any problems.

The clinician looks at Rodney. Rodney looks down at the floor and is quiet. The clinician allows about 15 seconds of silence. The rest of the family remains quiet too.

Clinician: *Rodney, you seem pretty quiet. Do you have something you might want to share?*

Rodney remains silent but glances at his parents.

Mother (after a pause): *During the past month or so he missed some school. He said he didn't feel good.*

Clinician (wondering whether a connection between a school stress and the fighting at home can be made): *Rodney, I know this might be hard to talk about, but it's important to know what's going on at school. Can you tell us a little more?*

With gentle coaxing and encouragement from his parents and the clinician, Rodney reveals that he is being bullied at school during recess. He has not told the teacher because he felt she would tell his father, and he does not want to disappoint his father, who has always urged the boys to be "tough."

Clinician (in acknowledgment of Rodney's feelings, paraphrases his story and attempts to help him express his feelings): *Rodney, thank you for sharing this. You've been through a lot. You had to see this bully every day. You couldn't tell the teachers or Mom or Dad. How did this make you feel?*

Rodney tells the family that he felt scared and sad. He restates again that he didn't want to disappoint his father because he is not fighting the bully. He feels his father might be angry with him.

Rodney: *Sometimes I don't want to go to school.*

Clinician (acknowledging Rodney's feelings again in an attempt to encourage elaboration): *So when you do go to school and then come home, you must feel pretty upset.*

Rodney: *Alex knows about the bully. When I come home, Alex teases me about being bullied and calls me a "wimp." Then I get mad at him and really want to beat him up.*

Father: *You never told us this.*

Rodney: *I didn't want to tell you. I thought you'd get mad at me. I made Alex promise he wouldn't tell.*

Mother: *This breaks my heart.*

Clinician: *It must be hard to hear this, but it helps all of us understand why the boys are fighting.*

When discussing the goal, keep the family focused on the goal. Families often fall back to "problem talk."

Father: *Sometimes I just think that if I took a firm stand and told the boys to stop fighting, that would end all of this.*

Mother: *I just don't know if I can take any more of this.*

Clinician: *I understand your feelings of frustration, but we have come a long way in this meeting by focusing on the family's goal about life at home and the bullying situation at school. Let's not focus on the past, but on the future.*

Step 3: Working With the Family

Working with the family, the "therapeutic" phase of the interview, consists mainly of the clinician facilitating changes in family behaviors and helping family members develop solutions. The clinician can make suggestions when necessary and appropriate. This step has 4 elements: (1) identifying family strengths, support systems, and past successes; (2) engaging the family in developing a plan of action; (3) suggesting interventions/offering advice; and (4) assigning homework tasks (Box 16.7).

> **Box 16.7. Working With the Family: Allow 20 to 25 Minutes for This Step[a]**
> 1. Identify family strengths, support systems, and past successes.
> 2. Engage the family in developing a plan of action and encourage collaboration.
> 3. Suggest interventions/advice.
> 4. Assign homework tasks.
> _____
> [a]These time limits are only approximations.

Identifying Family Strengths, Support Systems, and Past Successes

Families often become so involved with the problem that they forget their strengths, support systems, or past successes. The clinician's job is to help the family rediscover and use these strengths and supports effectively. *"We've discussed the concern enough and I understand it. Now I'd like to ask you about things that each of you individually and as a family have done that makes you feel good about each other and/or has helped the family be happier together."*

Case Study 16.1 (continued)

Clinician (pointing out the family's strengths): *I want to remind you that you are a family with many strengths. You are caring and very supportive of each other. Coming here and talking with each other make that clear. You also have support from relatives.*

Father: *That's good to hear.*

Clinician (searching for other successes): *What else have you done in the past that worked and might be tried again?*

The family recalled that, when the boys had been enrolled in after-school sports, they were very happy and got along well.

Clinician (looking for more specific supports): *Who provided transportation?*

Father (identifying another support): *A neighbor whose son also plays sports.*

Engaging the Family in Developing a Plan of Action and Encouraging Collaboration

The clinician helps the family develop a plan of action that facilitates a change in the family's behaviors by combining its strengths, past successes, new insights, and goals. The plan requires the cooperation of all family members.

Case Study 16.1 (continued)

Clinician (reminding the family of its cooperation in the meeting): *You've shown that you are willing to work together. What can you do as a family that will help you achieve your goal?*

The mother states she will listen to the boys when they come to her with their problems and will not automatically send them to their father. The father states that he too could spend more time listening to the boys and that he will not be so insistent that they be "tough." He also feels he had relied too much on his own father's advice.

Clinician: *Do you think explaining this to the boys' grandfather would help? Once he understands would he be supportive of you?*

The parents are not sure if the grandfather would understand and support them.

Clinician (to the boys): *What would you like to do instead of fighting?*

The boys state their wish to participate again in after-school sports.

Mother (identifying a strength): *The boys are good at sports. We let that slide. But when they play, they feel good and so do we.*

Clinician: *How can you make that happen?*

Father (demonstrating initiative and leadership): *I could speak with our neighbor again. Maybe we can take turns driving to ensure it really happens.*

Clinician: *How are you feeling about this?*

Father: *This all sounds good, but I'm not sure we can do all of this. It's not that easy.*

Clinician: *You have a right to be cautious, but your goal is clear and realistic. Is everyone willing to cooperate?*

The family's mood brightens a bit, and the family members state their willingness.

Suggesting Interventions/Offering Advice

Suggestions and advice are helpful if the family
- Wants them and is ready to listen and attempt change
- Understands them
- Is prepared to try them
- Agrees to them as a family
- Feels they fit the problem and its family values
- Has the capabilities and resources to carry them out

The clinician can also be directive if the family is ready to change and can suggest specific interventions aimed at the family as a whole and/or at individuals. The PCP needs to be careful in how directive to be. The PCP should help the family take a first step (eg, a very simple first step to its goal). Sometimes parents request specific advice. The clinician should not rush too fast with advice. The family should first try to construct its own solutions. The advice that the clinician gives must respect the family hierarchy, fit the family's coping ability, and support its goals.

When offering advice, the clinician must avoid 3 common pitfalls.

1. Failure to "join" with the family and gain its trust
2. Failure to understand the concern or goal within the family context
3. Failure to understand that the family is not ready to accept, or act on, the advice at this time

Clinicians often fall into these pitfalls because they feel pressured to "do something" quickly (eg, write a prescription) and "fix" the child's symptoms, thus they ignore family issues and influences.

Case Study 16.1 (continued)

Mother: *We need your advice about the bullying at school.*

The clinician could offer to call the school, but she wants the family to take the initiative to act, create its own solutions, and feel more empowered. She does offer some advice.

Clinician: *I suggest that you call the teacher tomorrow and tell her the situation. Ask to arrange a meeting with her, the school counselor, and the two of you (looking at both parents). Rodney should be there too. The meeting should take place after school in a quiet, private room. The school has a good policy regarding bullying. Both the bully and Rodney will get help and support. I will call later, if necessary. Do you think that would be helpful?*

The parents thank the clinician. Rodney looks grateful and relieved.

Clinician: *Rodney, how does this sound to you?*

Rodney: *Okay.*

Clinician (complimenting the family and supporting them): *I like the idea of signing up the boys for after-school sports.*

Father: *Maybe Grandpa could help out here. He loves watching the boys play sports.*

Assigning Homework Tasks

At the end of a family meeting, the clinician can assign the family a homework task of practicing the new tasks/behaviors/interactions. If these changes are to become the new reality, they must take place in the home, not just in the meeting. Because changing behavioral patterns takes time, practice, work, reminders, and encouragement, having an assigned task must appeal to all members. They must understand that a task requires real work and mutual support. The task should be geared to the goal that has been discussed.

Case Study 16.1 (continued)

Clinician: *I'd like to suggest a homework task for the family. But first let's briefly review the goals you would like to discuss in your home family meetings. One of the best things you did here today was to listen to each other. You have stated that was something you want to do, so I'd like to suggest a weekly family meeting. If you can't do it weekly, twice a month would be okay. Try it and see how it works.*

The clinician explains how to conduct a family meeting at home and gives the family a handout with more details. For more details, see Chapter 30.

Clinician (getting feedback from the family): *Do you think this might help?*

Mother: *We'll try it.*

Father: *It can't hurt.*

The boys shrug their shoulders.

Step 4: Concluding the Session

Concluding the session in a controlled, non-abrupt manner conveys a sense of order, professionalism, and clinician leadership and also gives the family members time to compose themselves and to consider final thoughts, feelings, and questions. The 6 elements of the concluding step are (1) making a transition to the conclusion, (2) summarizing the meeting, (3) letting the family respond, (4) getting family feedback, (5) scheduling the next visit, and (6) complimenting and thanking the family (Box 16.8).

Box 16.8. Concluding the Session: Allow 10 Minutes for This Step[a]

1. Make the transition to the conclusion.
2. Summarize the meeting.
3. Let the family respond.
4. Get family feedback.
5. Schedule the next visit.
6. Compliment and thank the family.

---
[a]These time limits are only an approximation.

Making the Transition to the Conclusion

The clinician must watch the time and allow sufficient time to conclude the meeting. The clinician's manner of making the transition to the conclusion tells the family that the meeting is ending. The clinician should be sure that this transition is stated on a complimentary note. He or she initiates the transition with a phrase, change of voice, and/or action. For example, he or she might state, *"It has been a good meeting. It's coming to a close; let's begin to wrap things up at this time."*

Case Study 16.1 (continued)

Clinician (glancing at the clock): *I see it's almost time to end our session.*

Summarizing the Meeting

The clinician uses the summarization to highlight and clarify the essential aspects of the meeting. The family is better able to remember the relevant aspects if they are condensed into a few succinct, clear statements. When this is done, the family is also more likely to respond with any remaining questions and comments. In addition, a clear summary conveys that the clinician has heard the family's concerns and that he or she respects and understands them. Finally, summarizing should always convey a sense of achievement and hope.

Case Study 16.1 (continued)

Clinician: *Let me take just a few minutes to summarize things, and then I'd like to hear from you. You came here because the boys were fighting. As we discussed, a combination of factors has kept the problem going. No one is to blame. You've demonstrated some real strengths, like your commitment to work together and your willingness to change your behaviors. You have supportive relatives and a helpful neighbor. You've come up with some excellent solutions, such as changing your responses to the boys, arranging a school meeting, providing after-school sports, sharing the driving, and even asking the boys' grandfather to help out. I've also suggested the family meetings at home. That's a lot. Congratulations, this is impressive and shows how caring and competent you are. Have I summarized this correctly? Let me hear what you think?*

Letting the Family Respond

The family members will invariably have final thoughts and questions. They need time and need to feel that they have "permission" to voice their thoughts and feelings without being criticized. The clinician invites each member of the family to speak. Members may wish to speak to the clinician, to the whole family, or to an individual. The responses also give the family a chance to hear how each member feels about the meeting (eg, *"Being here really helped."* or *"This meeting was a waste of time."*).

Getting Family Feedback

If the family does not offer feedback about the meeting, the clinician should ask (the family and/or individuals) if the meeting was useful or satisfying, (eg, *"How did this meeting help or not help?"* or *"Did we address your concerns satisfactorily?"*). If anyone expresses a doubt, the clinician should respectfully ask him or her to elaborate.

Case Study 16.1 (continued)

Clinician (asking an open-ended question): *What questions or comments do you have for me or for other members of the family?*

Mother to the family: *I am glad we came here.*

Rodney: *Will the bully bother me again?*

The clinician looks over to the father to give him the chance to respond and to demonstrate his support for his son.

Father: *Rodney, don't worry. We are going do everything possible to take care of that. And I want to tell both of you* (looking at the boys) *that you can always come and talk to me, and I will not tell you to just tough it out.*

Sometimes when families express feelings, such as affection, remorse, pride, or sorrow, they want to touch each other (eg, kissing, hugging, squeezing the shoulder, holding hands, patting the back), but they may feel hesitant or unsure about whether doing so is "okay." The clinician should show sensitivity to these special moments. If appropriate, he or she might encourage this demonstration by remaining silent or by saying something like, *"Show him how much you care."*

Scheduling the Next Visit and Updating the Family's Progress

The clinician schedules follow-up visits at this time. The first should be scheduled 2 to 3 weeks later, if possible. Subsequent visits can be scheduled farther apart as progress is made. The follow-up visit provides the clinician with information on how the family is doing and on whether the prior meeting was successful. Families need the follow-up visit to discuss their progress or lack thereof and to get feedback and encouragement from the clinician. If a family isn't progressing, it needs additional intervention and support. The clinician should use this meeting to determine if he or she missed something or moved too quickly. The family might also have a new problem that requires the PCP's attention. Scheduling a follow-up visit(s) also demonstrates the clinician's ongoing interest in and support for the family.

If there is no progress after several visits, the PCP should discuss in a no-blame/no-shame manner, *"I sense I'm not able to help you resolve your issues. Maybe I missed something or moved too fast. Maybe the family felt it was too much."* The PCP should let the family respond and take cues from the family's response in order to determine the next step (eg, continue sessions with a different approach, end the sessions, or consider a referral). The PCP should always be available if and when the family wants to return or wants referral information.

Case Study 16.1 (continued)

Clinician: *I'd like to schedule a follow-up meeting in 2 to 3 weeks. Will that work for you? If anything comes up before that, please give me a call.*

Complimenting and Thanking the Family

Compliments should be offered in a genuine and generous manner that recognizes the family's positive attributes and strengths. Compliments help the family "reframe" others, itself, or its internal interactions by replacing a negative perception of others or a negative self-image with a positive one.

Case Study 16.1 (continued)

Clinician: *This has been an effective meeting. Your commitment to one another is very apparent. Look at all you accomplished today. In this sense it has been a good meeting. Each of you contributed to the success of this meeting. Rodney, you were very brave in sharing your story about school. Alex, you said you want to be friends with Rodney. That was very kind. And* (to the father) *I think it was very important that you told the boys they can come and talk to you and that they don't always need to be tough. And* (to the mother) *sharing your feelings with Rodney about spanking him was also very significant. Thank you for coming in. I look forward to our next visit.*

Chapter 17

After the Interview: The Post-Interview Phase and Follow-up

*A*fter the interview, the pediatric care professional (PCP) has several tasks in the post-interview phase, the time the clinician uses (a) to review the quality of the meeting, (b) to assess his or her own feelings, (c) to prepare for the next meeting, and (d) to determine a termination point. Subsequently, follow-up visits represent the only way for the PCP to measure the success of the meetings and to ascertain the family's status. The PCP must realize that, at some point in the clinician–family relationship, the PCP and the family must terminate the meetings when the goals have been achieved or when a referral is needed. If the sessions are not helpful, the PCP must get family feedback and remind them that the family does have strengths in solving the family challenges, but that they may not yet be ready or they might work with another professional. The PCP should compliment them on their efforts and consider a referral. (See Chapter 31.)

In the post-interview phase, the clinician reviews the quality of the meeting. Questions the clinician can ask himself or herself are listed below. In general, the clinician wants to know the following: Was the meeting a success or failure? What worked? What failed? If something failed, how can it be fixed? The clinician needs input from the family to obtain the best answers to these questions.

ASSESSING THE EFFECTIVENESS OF THE MEETING AND THE FAMILY'S SATISFACTION

- Did the clinician respect the presenting concern and stay focused on it, or did he or she change the focus without the family's invitation, consent, or awareness? For example, a family complains that the son's attention-deficit/ hyperactivity disorder problem is causing family conflict; however, the clinician presumes that the family conflict is really caused by the parents' marital tension and chooses to focus on that instead. The family understandably will feel disrespected and dissatisfied by this unannounced, premature, and possibly incorrect shift. If marital tension is present, it will usually be revealed in a later visit as the clinician gains the family's trust and explores the family context.

- Were the family's goals specific and realistic? If not, did the clinician help them define and negotiate more specific and realistic goals? For example, the family's goal may be *"We want to be a happy family,"* which is vague and unrealistic. The PCP must then help the family define and negotiate a more specific and realistic goal (eg, *"We'd like to have two pleasant evenings each week doing something together, such as talking, playing board games and cards, or watching TV."*)

- Did the clinician explain the purpose of the family meeting? Does the family understand? Did the family members "accept" the idea of a family meeting?

- Was everyone involved in the session? Did the PCP form an alliance with each member of the family ("touch" each member) and encourage his or her participation?

- Did the clinician identify the hierarchy and family structure (eg, leadership, coalitions, and boundaries)?

- Did the clinician help the members develop new interactions? Did the clinician engage the family in a cooperative effort? Was he or she too directive?

- Was the session comfortable and orderly? Did the PCP make it "safe" for all family members to express themselves without fear of ridicule or disapproval? Was the meeting time-efficient?

- Was it necessary to impose rules for the session or to change the seating? Did the clinician demonstrate appropriate leadership?

- Does the family appear satisfied? Do the members feel some progress has been made? How does the PCP know? Did he or she ask them, *"Are you all in agreement? Would you like to keep meeting? Are you satisfied how things are now?"* The PCP should help the family decide the next step in addressing their issues.

- Does the family seem willing to return? Gauging its willingness can be difficult. Even a statement such as, *"Yes, we'll come back,"* does not guarantee its return.

THE CLINICIAN'S SELF-ASSESSMENT OF HIS/HER "PERFORMANCE"

The clinician should ask himself or herself some questions about his or her own actions and emotional response to the family.

- How does the clinician feel about the family? What were his or her positive or negative feelings about it?
- Did the clinician convey these feelings to the family, either intentionally or unintentionally? How?
- What would the clinician do differently in the next meeting?
- Did the clinician identify too closely with either the family or an individual member? Did he or she thus lose objectivity or effectiveness? Did he or she form a coalition with a parent or child?
- Does the clinician have a "rescue fantasy," a wish to "save" the family, that caused him or her to rush in too fast with advice or to make impossible promises?
- Does the clinician want to see the family again?
- Would the clinician prefer that this family not return? If not, what should he or she do? This may be a way of thinking about a referral. The referral suggestion should be made in a way that does not suggest to the family that they are not wanted anymore, but rather as a way of helping them.

PREPARING FOR THE NEXT MEETING

The clinician prepares for the next meeting by asking more questions of himself or herself.

- Does the clinician think that his or her initial impression/hypothesis needs to be revised?
- What other information does the clinician think is still needed?
- Should the clinician invite other members if it might be helpful in assisting the family to develop its goals?
- Should the clinician consider making a referral?
- The clinician should make a plan for the next visit (eg, invite another member, add more structure and order, encourage more communication between certain members, or direct the family focus to a particular issue).

REVIEWING FOR THE NEXT MEETING

Several helpful tasks that assist the clinician's preparation for the next meeting are given below.

- The clinician can revise the original hypothesis after the first meeting when more is learned about the family. For example, what might first appear as a parenting disagreement about discipline now seems to be the symptom of alcoholism instead. The parents avoid confronting the drinking problem by maintaining their parenting disagreements. The symptom (parents arguing) operates as a way to maintain the family balance and function.

- With the family's consent, the clinician can obtain copies of past individual or family evaluations, school records, or any other information that might prove helpful in understanding the family. A record of attempted interventions and outcomes often proves very helpful.
- The clinician can speak with a consultant or a colleague to get a second opinion or to seek guidance for the next meeting.
- The clinician should dictate or write a chart note. He or she must document the visit for both medical–legal and billing purposes (see Chapter 32); to record confidential, important information; and to summarize the visit. Reviewing the notes before the next meeting helps the clinician remember the pertinent points and organize his or her approach.

FOLLOW-UP MEETINGS

In the busy practice setting, the clinician may need 2 meetings to carry out a complete initial interview. The first visit entails engaging and understanding the family, and the second entails working with the family. Then, shorter follow-up visits are used to gauge the success of the meetings and to show support for the family efforts.

Follow-up meetings

- Provide the clinician with a better understanding of the family's ability to develop its goals. Every meeting reveals more information about the family's communication patterns and adaptability.
- Reveal the efficacy of the clinician and the treatment plan. Follow-up visits are the only way for the clinician to measure the success of the meeting. They provide feedback about the clinician's abilities.

Steps of Follow-up Meetings

Follow-up meetings are usually shorter than the initial meeting, but follow a similar sequence of steps: (1) engaging the family, (2) updating the family's situation, (3) working with the family in their present situation, and (4) concluding the session.

- **Engaging the family.** Follow-up visits start with a welcoming, friendly greeting to put the family at ease (eg, *"It's good to see you all again. Thank you for making the effort to get together again."*). If a family member is attending for the first time, the clinician needs to introduce himself or herself, welcome the new member, and determine this individual's relationship to and role in the family. Questions for assessing this include, *"What is your relationship to Timmy (the child)?" "Do you live with the family?"* and *"What is your role in the family (eg, caretaking responsibilities, decision-making)?"*

- **Understanding the family's situation.** This phase should begin with open-ended questions (eg, *"Tell me how things have been going since our last visit."*). The follow-up visit provides more information about the family in several ways.
  — Family meetings stir up feelings that remind the family of other issues; in the follow-up visit the family may wish to focus on these feelings or issues instead of on the initial complaint. When this happens, the clinician should respect the family's wish and should explore the new issue for a short time. Then the clinician must help the family determine what is more important at this time—the initial complaint or this present issue. For example, a family's original complaint might be poor family communication (*"We yell and scream all the time."*), but at the follow-up visit its new issue might be the family's disappointment about the child's recent report card (*"He's failed math."*). The clinician needs to provide some leadership and help the family decide which to discuss. The other issue can also be addressed at another meeting.
  — In a follow-up visit, the family may feel more comfortable and thus may talk more openly. Beginning with an open-ended question allows the members to reveal new information, if they wish. The family also may want to review or clarify certain aspects of the previous meeting.
    During the interval between visits, the family may have experienced an unexpected event—either negative or positive—that it may want to discuss at the meeting. If the family's reply is, *"We're not doing so well,"* the clinician should first acknowledge those feelings. He or she might say, *"I'm sorry to hear that. Let's take a few minutes and review what happened. Were you all clear about or in agreement with what happened at the last meeting? What do you think has been difficult since the last meeting? What have you achieved?"*
  — When things don't go well for the family and/or it doesn't make progress, the clinician must also consider whether the suggestions that he or she made were accurate, timely, or clear. The clinician can convey this by saying, *"Maybe I suggested something before I really understood the situation."* or *"Maybe I didn't make myself clear in our last meeting."* The clinician should not label the family as "noncompliant," "resistant," or "difficult." Instead, the PCP should explore the reasons for the family's reluctance to adhere to its plans.
  — Is the family doing better? If the family reports *"We are doing better,"* the clinician should ask the members to elaborate with specifics. Good news and progress should never be taken for granted or minimized.

These are the "victories" that the family wants, needs, and is working for. The clinician can ask the following questions:

- *"What is better?"*
- *"What are you doing now?"*
- *"How did you do it?"*
- *"Did the family cooperate?"*
- *"Does everyone share this feeling?*

- **Working with the family in their present situation.** In this part of the interview, the clinician helps the family further develop or refine solutions. If the family is "doing better" (changing the interactions, expectations, roles, or perceptions), it might be content to "rest" at this point. The clinician can help the family members decide if they want to "work" or to "rest" and should support their decision. If the family wants to work, the clinician might use the scaling question: *"So, let me ask you a question. At the last meeting you said you all felt you were at a 6 in terms of doing well. What would you have to do to go from a 6 to a 7?"* Together the family can devise a few strategies. See Chapter 24 for more examples of the solution-oriented interview.

  If this visit is planned to be the last, the clinician should remind the family so that they can prepare to say goodbye.

- **Concluding the meeting.** The clinician should leave 10 minutes for the conclusion in the plan for the meeting. The clinician concludes the meeting by providing a brief summary to help the family remember its accomplishments and the tasks ahead (*"Let me review what we've done here today."*). This synopsis is especially helpful for the discouraged family or one that has difficulty following through and accomplishing its goals. The clinician should also ask the family members how they feel about the sessions and should give them time to respond (*"What are your thoughts and feelings about the meeting? What helped? What didn't help?"*). The PCP should always find genuine reasons to compliment the family and leave them with a sense of hope and competence. (*"You've done good work in these meetings. Thank you for all your hard work. This is great, you have really achieved your goals and you have accomplished a great deal as a family. You should be proud of yourselves."*).

Scheduling the Follow-up Visits

The clinician should give the family an idea of how many follow-up visits he or she thinks are necessary (*"Let's plan on three or four visits. We can schedule more visits if necessary."*).

As a general guide, if the complete initial interval requires 2 sessions, those should be scheduled as close to one another as possible and should take place no more than 1 to 2 weeks apart. The first actual follow-up visit should be scheduled 1 to 3 weeks after the completed initial interview(s).

Subsequent follow-up visits should be scheduled at increasingly longer inter-vals—up to 2 to 3 months apart—depending on the family's progress and the clinician's judgment.

CHOOSING A TERMINATION POINT FOR THE MEETINGS

The purpose of family meetings is to make the family competent enough so it no longer needs the clinician's help. At some point, the clinician and fam-ily will realize that the family is not dependent on the clinician any more; it is capable of problem-solving/goal accomplishment on its own. The family members have achieved their goal. When the family and the clinician make this realization, they should choose a time together for terminating the meet-ings. Ideally, the clinician should schedule a final meeting because this meet-ing allows time for the clinician and the family to express their final feelings and thoughts and to say good-bye. The clinician reminds the family that he or she is always available. If the PCP is the pediatrician or nurse practitioner, he or she will still have an ongoing relationship with the family.

Below are listed a few different situations that signal that the time to termi-nate the meetings has arrived.

- In the course of a routine follow-up session, the clinician and/or the family sense that the family is competent and that it doesn't need to come back. Suddenly, this routine session becomes the final one. In this case, the clinician should voice this idea and should let the family respond (unless they have already voiced it). If the members agree, the clinician should provide enough time in that meeting for all family members to share their final thoughts.

- The clinician and the family have agreed to a specific number of meet-ings. If the family members have agreed to 3 meetings, the clinician should remind them at the end of the second meeting that the next visit (the third) is their last scheduled meeting. When the third visit begins, the clinician can remind them that this visit is the final meeting (*"Before we begin, let me remind you that this is our last scheduled visit."*). The clinician should always allow a few minutes at the end of the meeting for both the family and the clinician to answer questions, to share final thoughts, and to say good-bye. The clinician should always offer the option of more visits if the family feels it needs or wants more. This is very reassuring. It should feel welcome to return in the future as necessary. The clinician can suggest more meetings if he or she feels that the family has not yet achieved its goal.

- Sometimes in the final meeting the clinician senses the family wants and needs more meetings, or the family indicates a continued need or desire to continue them. In this situation, the clinician might say, *"Although this is our last scheduled visit, we can schedule more if you would like."* or *"I think that one or two more visits would be very helpful."*

- The family's goal is achieved before the final scheduled visit. For example, the clinician and the family initially scheduled 4 visits, but by the end of the third visit the family has demonstrated so much adaptability and growth that the fourth visit appears unnecessary. The clinician might raise the issue while still offering the family the full number of agreed-on visits. He or she might say, *"You seem to be doing so well that the fourth visit may not be necessary. I still would be very happy to see you at the next scheduled visit, or we can schedule it at a later date. But I need to hear what you think."*

- Sometimes the family raises the issue of a final meeting. A family member may say, *"Doctor, we feel we have made progress in these three meetings and don't need a fourth visit."* The clinician should agree with the family, if he or she thinks the family has made sufficient progress, by saying, *"I agree. We don't need the fourth meeting, but I am always available if you want to return."*

    If the clinician feels the family needs the fourth visit, he or she should be frank yet supportive. He or she could say, *"I agree that you've made real progress, but I think that one more visit would be helpful. We can schedule it for a longer interval. Is that okay with you?"*

Chapter 18

Family Interviewing: 3 Brief Case Studies

*B*efore a family meeting, some pediatric care professionals (PCPs) find it helpful to review several basic principles. Four examples are listed below followed by 3 brief case studies.

1. **Family membership.** Who are the members of the family? Do they live in the same house? What do they do? What is the hierarchy? Do they have extended families?
2. **Family balance or stability.** How does the family maintain emotional and functional stability? What are the interpersonal processes that allow the family to function in a healthy way? What are the roles and actions of the family members?
3. **Family adaptability.** How does the family adapt and cope with sudden change, loss, or stress? How do members interact in the face of change? Do they shift their positions and roles, change their expectations and behavior, or adapt to changing family relationships?
4. **The symptom(s) in a family–relationship context.** Because the child's symptom is influenced by the family–psychosocial context, the physician must examine it by asking questions: What is the significance of the symptom to the family? What purpose does it serve? How does the family affect the child's symptom? How does the child's symptom affect the family? Understanding the relationship between the symptom and the family context reveals important diagnostic and therapeutic information. For example, a child's recurrent headaches may have begun when his father suffered a severe stroke.

CASE STUDY 18.1: A 6-YEAR-OLD BOY WITH ENURESIS

A Child-Centered Problem Recurs or Intensifies Despite Multiple Symptom-Centered Interventions

A mother brings her boy in for bed-wetting. The clinician performs a physical examination, orders a urinalysis, and suggests several interventions (medication, bladder-stretching exercises, and sleep alarms). At the next meeting, the mother reports that she and her husband haven't adhered to the suggestions because they disagree with each other about them, especially the use of medication and/or sleep alarms. The clinician then suggests that the parents try withholding fluid after 6:00 pm and waking the boy to use the bathroom before they go to bed. The clinician asks that both parents come to the next meeting.

Both parents come in 2 weeks but state that they find that agreeing to carry out this second set of instructions is difficult for them. The clinician suggests, *"Put your differences aside for the boy's sake."* At the subsequent visit, the parents reveal that they are still at odds about treatment and state that, *"The wetting is causing a lot of family tension."* The boy's schoolmates know that he has a bed-wetting problem and teased him at school, and now the boy refuses to attend. The mother and father take turns staying at home, convincing the boy to go, and then driving him to school when he agrees to go. The boy is sad and tearful, and the parents have become even more upset with him and with each other.

At this point, the clinician decides to adopt a family systems perspective and to explore the family context so that he can help them resolve the parental disagreements and the boy's enuresis. After explaining the purpose for using the family meeting approach, he asks the parents about their beliefs about enuresis, their family health histories, and their own experiences growing up with their parents ("parenting histories").

The father reveals that he suffered from enuresis as a child and states that his parents *"beat it out of me."* He didn't like it, but *"it worked for me."* He feels his son *"should learn to control it like I did."* He doesn't spank his son, but he readily shows his displeasure.

The mother reports that her parents, who were indulgent, raised her by reasoning with her and showing affection and that they never spanked her. She tends to *"make excuses"* for her son and even hides his wet underpants from the father, only adding to the family tension. Although the mother wants to try the interventions, her husband refuses. The clinician helps the parents cooperate and develop more effective strategies.

The clinician explains the following:

- The influence of the parents' backgrounds on their differing beliefs and parenting styles
- The effects of their conflict, which is prolonging the enuresis and affecting the boy's self-esteem and school life
- The effects of the conflict, which is causing family tension and affecting their relationship with each other
- Explaining enuresis in a way that removes blame from the boy and that shows that his symptom is still within normal variation
- Ways to change their behaviors

The parents respond in the following ways:

- The father agrees not to show his anger.
- The father agrees to try the interventions for 1 month.
- The mother agrees not to "protect" the boy by hiding the underpants.
- They agree to contact their son's teacher, who promises to try to stop the teasing.
- They insist that their son return to school.

The enuresis gradually resolves, even though the boy has occasional brief relapses. The parents still disagree on some aspects of parenting but do agree more often. Their arguments occur less frequently; when they do occur, they are less intense.

CASE STUDY 18.2: A 4-YEAR-OLD GIRL WITH TANTRUMS

The Parent Ignores the Clinician's Advice

A divorced father reports that his daughter's tantrums, which occur both at home and in public, are extremely *"embarrassing, because people think I'm abusing her."* She always asks for toys and candy; when her father refuses, she has a "meltdown." The clinician suggests that the father use extinction techniques and says, *"Just don't pay any attention. Let her scream all she wants. When she realizes that she's not getting your attention or the goodies, the tantrums will subside. You can praise her when she shows improvement of any kind."* During the visit, the girl plays with toys and draws pictures. She is well-behaved.

At the follow-up visit, the father reports that the *"meltdowns are the same."* When asked about his attempts to use the technique, he states that he stopped after 2 attempts because *"people still think I'm abusing her."* He appears downcast and helpless. The clinician decides to shift to a family–social context to understand the problem better and the father's sadness. She explains the purpose of a family meeting and the involvement of the family context of the problem, not just the child's symptom.

The clinician then inquires about the father's ex-wife and about their relationship. He reports that his former wife had moved to another city and that the girl visits her mother only one weekend a month. The relationship between the father and mother is *"cold."* The father then falls silent. After about 20 seconds of silence, the clinician reflects, *"You seem pretty sad and discouraged."* The father nods without making eye contact. She then asks, *"Have you been under any other stresses recently?"* The father states that his career involves long hours and frequent travel. He feels guilty about the divorce and the separation from his daughter.

He wants to be a good father when he is with his daughter. He fears that saying "no" or ignoring her demands will harm her self-esteem or that *"maybe she won't love me."* He also admits that, at the same time, he is becoming increasingly resentful toward her because *"every outing is spoiled."* This attitude leads to feeling even guiltier because of his resentment. He says, *"I'm really a bad father."*

During this visit, the girl plays quietly for a while. Later however, she begins pestering her father and interrupts him frequently. He pauses to respond to each interruption and tries to reason with her or to promise her ice cream if she behaves, all to no avail.

The clinician assures the father that he is not a bad parent and tells him very emphatically that he is a very devoted father and that he is doing a very good job as a single, hardworking dad. However, she explains, his guilt makes it difficult for him to respond appropriately to his daughter's tantrums. The clinician points out that tantrums are normal behavior for children of this age, but that his daughter's have intensified to a severe level, which is straining the parent–child relationship.

The clinician is directive. In this case, being directive is okay, as it seems it is needed. She encourages the father to say "no" without feeling guilty and to set limits. She gives him suggestions for what he can do when the girl acts up again.

The clinician encourages the father to develop his own solutions as well. She adds that setting limits will not cause the father to lose his daughter's love or to diminish her self-esteem. She also addresses the father's social context and asks him to consider ways in which to revive his social life.

At the next visit, the father reports that things are a bit better. He has called his ex-wife and explained the situation. They have agreed to change the visitation schedule so that he has more time to himself. Because the girl's mother wants to see her daughter more often, this gesture alone has improved the parents' relationship. This improvement in parental communication appears to exert a good influence on the girl. Both parents use the same approach to respond to the tantrums. Her tantrums occur less frequently, and she is not as whiny or irritable. The father is able to enjoy time with his daughter more than before. Over the next few visits, the situation remains stable.

CASE STUDY 18.3: A 9-YEAR-OLD GIRL WITH CHRONIC ABDOMINAL PAIN

Child Presents as the "Symptomatic Patient" or the "Identified Patient" of a Disturbed Family System

A mother makes an appointment for her daughter who suffers from chronic abdominal pain. The clinician takes a detailed history of the complaint and performs a physical examination. He finds no cause, so he refers the girl to a gastroenterologist who, after carrying out various tests and procedures, finds no organic etiology. The clinician prescribes an over-the-counter antacid medication.

The mother calls again, saying that the pain is still present and that *"the girl's grandmother is very worried."* This statement prompts the clinician to suggest a family meeting that includes the child's grandmother. When mother, father, daughter, and grandmother arrive, the clinician explains the purpose of the meeting. After asking about recent family changes, he finds that the pain began shortly after the grandmother moved in with the family.

The clinician takes a family history. The parents are in good physical and mental health but the grandmother has ulcers, which are a daily topic of conversation. The grandmother complains about her ulcers and dietary restrictions, so the mother feels obligated to give her a lot of attention, including rides to the doctor's office and to the drugstore. In her free time she works at her part-time job. She constantly feels tired and takes naps whenever she can.

The father has increased his work hours to help pay for the care and living expenses of the grandmother. Often he leaves the house at 6:00 am and does not return until after dinner, leaving him with no time to spend with his daughter. Because the family routines and relationships are disrupted, the girl almost seems to be ignored by her parents. When she is alone with her grandmother, she is expected to keep her company and to take care of her. The grandmother, alarmed when the girl experienced abdominal pain because *"ulcers run in the family,"* had suggested to the parents the idea for the extensive medical evaluations.

The clinician is able to identify the dynamics influencing the daughter's abdominal pain. He explains how the family's changes have affected the relationships and how these changes are most likely contributing to the girl's symptoms. The family responds appreciatively to this explanation, and the clinician encourages them to develop a new interactional plan at home.

At the next meeting, the family shares its plan. The grandmother discusses her ulcers less frequently and does not mention them at all with her granddaughter; the mother enrolls the grandmother in the senior center 3 days a week. During that time, the mother and daughter spend time together talking, doing errands, cooking, or walking the dog. The parents make all decisions about their daughter's health care. When the girl is alone with her grandmother, they participate in activities that they both enjoy, such as reading, baking, or watching TV. However, the girl's pain continues. The clinician urges them to be patient and to keep doing the same things.

By the subsequent visit, the girl's pain has decreased in frequency and intensity. The family, who is still adjusting to the grandmother living with them, finds that the plans do not always work. Still, the family members feel that they are doing better. *"We can live with things now,"* they say.

SECTION D SUMMARY

This section has described a detailed overview of the 4 steps of a family interview: engaging the family, understanding the family and its concerns, working with the family, and concluding the interview. It has also described the post-interview phase and follow-up visits. What happens after the initial meeting carries as much importance as the initial meeting itself. The clinician has several tasks. In the post-interview phase, he or she reviews the quality of the meeting, assesses his or her personal feelings, and plans for the next meeting. Follow-up visits are essential as they are the only way for the clinician to measure the success of the meetings and the family's status. Finally, as the series of family meetings eventually come to an end, the clinician must know how and when to end these meetings.

Many suggestions are offered, many more that can be used in a single interview, but in reality each PCP must pick and choose his or her questions and techniques for the interview. There is no single or "correct" way to interview a family. Each PCP develops his or her own style based on personal skills and preferences, the presenting problem, the family's coping abilities, communication patterns, the family–clinician relationship, and the time constraints of the office/clinic setting. Being aware of the steps of the interview and how to arrange follow-up visits make the family meetings organized, effective, satisfying, and time-efficient.

Skills Checklist

- Discuss the 4 steps of a family interview.
- Discuss the components of each step and discuss which components you might select for your interviews to best fit families in your practice/clinic.
- Discuss how you might organize and pace a family interview.
- Discuss the importance of the post-interview phase and follow-up phase.
- Discuss the components of these phases.

- Realize that an interview does not always proceed in a predictable sequence.
- Discuss what you might do if the meeting did not go well (for the family and/or for you).
- Discuss how to always leave the family with a sense of achievement.
- Discuss when you want to consider a referral.
- With a colleague, practice asking various questions. Set up a role-playing situation.

SUGGESTED READING

Alderfer MA, Fiese BG, Gold JI, et al. Evidence-based assessment in pediatric psychology family measures. *J Pediatr Psychol.* 2008;33(9):1046–1061; discussion 1062–1064

Allmond BW, Tanner JL. *The Family Is the Patient.* 2nd ed. Baltimore. MD: Williams & Wilkins; 1999

Brown JD, Wissow LS, Riley AW. Physician and patient characteristics associated with discussion of psychosocial health during pediatric primary care visits. *Clin Pediatr (Phila).* 2007;46(9):812–820

Campbell TL, McDaniel S. Conducting a family interview. In: Lipkin M, Putnam SM, Lazare AR, eds. *The Medical Interview.* New York, NY: Springer-Verlag; 1995:178–186

Coleman WL. *Family-Focused Behavioral Pediatrics.* Philadelphia, PA: Lippincott, Williams and Wilkins; 2001

Coleman WL. Family-focused pediatrics: a primary care family systems approach to psychosocial problems. *Curr Probl Pediatr Adolesc Health Care.* 2002;(32):260–305

Coleman WL. The first interview with a family. *Pediatr Clin North Am.* 1995;42(1):119–129

Corlett J, Twycross A. Negotiation of parental roles within family-centered care: a review of the research. *J Clin Nurs.* 2006;15(10):1308–1316

Josephson AM. Practice parameter for the assessment of the family. *J Am Acad Child Adolesc Psychiatry.* 2007;46(7):922–937

Korsch BM. *The Intelligent Patient's Guide to the Doctor Patient Relationship.* New York, NY: Oxford University Press; 1997

Ludwig S, Rostain A. Family function and dysfunction. In: Levine MD, Carey WB, Crocker AC, Coleman WL, Elias E, Feldman H, eds. *Developmental–Behavioral Pediatrics.* 4th ed. Philadelphia, PA: Elsevier; 2009

Marshall AJ, Harper-Jaques S. Depression and family relationships: ideas for healing. *J Fam Nurs.* 2008;14(1):56–73

Morrison J. *The First Interview.* New York, NY: Guilford Press; 1995

Weber T, McKeever JE, McDaniel SH. A beginner's guide to the problem-oriented first family interview. *Fam Process.* 1985;24:357–364

Conceptual Models of Family Interviewing With Case Studies

Virginia Satir—The Communication Model: Strategies to Improve Family Communication

*F*amily communication is one of the biggest challenges families face. One of the most frequent complaints from families is, *"We can't communicate."* Parents complain that children *"don't listen,"* and children complain that parents *"don't listen."* Everyone wants to be heard, yet nobody seems to listen (eg, the failure to accept another's position). Communication is a dynamic, interactive process that entails both functional listening and speaking. The most difficult aspect of family communication is the inability of family members to communicate their feelings clearly and effectively, especially love/affection, anger, or sadness. When family communication is problematic, strained relationships result.

The Satir model is based on several principles. Communication and behavioral interactional patterns are determined by a member's self-worth, place and role in the family, sense of attachment between parent and child, and biological determinants such as temperament and development.

Members' communication patterns may be functional or dysfunctional. Functional communication is clear and understandable in its expression of thoughts and feelings. One can accept responsibility for his or her actions. Differences between 2 members are viewed as an opportunity to learn, not as a threat.

Satir believed that functional communication promotes clarification, validation, intact self-esteem, negotiation, qualifying statements, and the ability to request feedback and to be receptive to feedback.

Dysfunctional communication is unclear, conflicting, and invalidating. This person is unable to clarify, restate, or modify meanings. He or she makes false assumptions and is unable to request, accept, or act on feedback. Differences are seen as threats.

A functional family member encountering a dysfunctional member would ask for clarification and qualification; however, the dysfunctional messenger will respond to this request with hostility, annoyance, and/or evasion, resulting in deterioration or termination of the encounter.

Satir further stated that both sender and receiver are responsible for clear and satisfying communication. Functional members, however, may have "flaws" if they too frequently generalize, question, and/or ask for feedback. Both parties must realize that perfect communication is not a reality because communication by its nature is never complete, but family members can strive for more complete and functional communication. Effective communication contributes greatly to each family member's self-esteem, self-image, sense of mastery, and personal validation (as parent, spouse, child, or sibling). Pediatric care professionals (PCPs) can support families and improve communication by revealing to them their own unique possibilities for changing their communication patterns and helping them to facilitate those changes.

Examples of communication problems (often leading to behavioral and emotional problems) follow:

Generalizing statements
- *"She is always ignoring me."*
- *"My husband never helps me with the work."*

Invalidating statements
- *"He's our designated bad child."*
- *"I feel I can never be a good parent."*

Others should understand how Mom feels
- *"You should know how I feel."*

Perceptions and opinions are complete and final
- *"No matter what you tell me, I won't change my mind."*

Mind reading
- *"I know what you're thinking."*

Family rules
- Family rules are unspoken, unconscious rules that impair communication and/or invalidate others.

The PCP must listen carefully and observe body language. He or she shares impressions and helps the family's communication by helping the family rephrase statements, clarify unclear messages, encourage feedback exchanges, eliminate false assumptions and generalizations, and encourage and support each member to speak honestly without fear of punishment or criticism. The PCP observes and interprets family communication and helps them improve their communication in the meeting.

Chapter 20

Family Communication Issues: Selected Examples of the Satir Model, Specific Interventions, and Case Studies

INEFFECTIVE LISTENING SKILLS: HOW TO TEACH LISTENING SKILLS

Listening and speaking are learned behaviors. The pediatric care professional (PCP) can help parents improve family communication by teaching listening and speaking skills. The communication style of the PCP is also a strong model. The case studies are centered on parent–child communication, but the skills can be applied to any family members (eg, parent–parent communication).

Parents Can Teach Listening Skills Early With These Techniques

- As children grow more verbal, parents can block out "listening times" when both child and parent are free from distractions, such as sitting quietly in a room (with the TV, computer games, and phones turned off and telephone answering machine turned on) or sharing a snack at bedtime. Car rides also provide excellent opportunities. The parent(s) can engage the child in a conversation about a topic of the child's choosing and then let the child do most of the talking.
- Reading to children, as young as 6 months, enhances listening. Parents should encourage children to comment and to ask questions about the material.

Parents Can Model Listening to Children Like They Themselves Want Their Children to Listen to Them

- Parents can use active listening. Children will learn to listen by observing how their parents listen. For example, active listening means actively responding with discernible verbal and nonverbal reactions to the speaker's thoughts and feelings (as represented by tone of voice, facial expression, and words). These listening skills include facial expressions that match the speaker's moods, eye contact, body posture, and 1- or 2-word responses (*"Uh-huh," "I see,"* or *"It sounds like you were feeling pretty good."*) or short summaries of what the child just said. Sitting at the child's level and making eye contact can help parents better detect the meanings and feelings portrayed by the child's words and facial expressions.
- Let children complete what they are saying. Sometimes parents react too quickly, interrupt, or say things that they don't really mean. Parents need to remember that children are just learning how to express themselves, a complex skill requiring time and practice, and that parental patience is crucial.

Parents Should Listen to Children When They Talk About Their Interests

Children love to talk about their adventures, fantasies, discoveries, and successes. They eagerly await the parent's response or feedback. Parents can do the following to encourage this interaction:

- Provide the time and encourage their children to talk about these things.
- Learn about the children's accomplishments in school, their after-school activities, their friends, and the popular culture (music, sports, fashions). This knowledge will provide much subject matter for discussion.
- Develop and discuss common interests with their children, which in turn motivates children to listen. For example, parents and children can watch TV and movies together and discuss their favorite movies, interests, TV shows, and activities.
- Tell their children about what they do at work. Children are interested in their parents' jobs and activities.
- If possible, take their children to work for a few hours.

Parents Can Appreciate the Child's Perspective

- Initially, parents should listen without judging or moralizing. A child communicates better when he or she feels that the parents respect his or her actions or viewpoints. Some parents find this difficult.
- Parents must learn when to talk and when to remain silent. For instance, if a child has a bad day at school, he or she may need time to settle down. Parents should wait until the child is ready to talk about the problem.

- Parents must understand the child's stage of language and social development so that the parent can help him or her learn to express himself or herself effectively and to use common courtesy (eg, *"May I?" "Excuse me," "Please,"* and *"Thank you.").*

Parents Can Recognize, Acknowledge, and Reward Good Listening Habits

Like other learned behaviors, listening is reinforced by positive feedback. *"I like the way you are looking at me and listening quietly."* Feedback is most effective when it is immediate, specific, and frequent (eg, at the end of a conversation, not hours or days later).

Parents Can Use Paraphrasing and Clarifying Statements When Listening

- Paraphrasing statements do the following:
  — Enhance the parents' understanding of what the child is saying.
  — Tell the child that he or she is heard.
  — Reduce the escalation of the child's anger (eg, *"So, what you are saying is that when no one plays with you, you feel upset."*).
  — Help children remember what they are saying.
- Parents can use clarifying statements for the following reasons:
  — Enhance their own understanding (eg, *"I'm not sure I understand."*).
  — Indicate that the parent is interested (eg, *"I want to know what you feel, but I need a little help."*).
  — Help the child improve his or her expressive language (eg, *"Do I understand that you mean...?"*).

Parents Can Teach Empathy by Listening With Empathy

Parents need to figure out the feelings that lie behind the child's words and that "drive" their behavior. Children feel strong emotions but have little experience expressing them or skills that are inadequate.

Child: *Are there big kids in school?*

The parent should make a supportive statement instead of a question, and the child can confirm, deny, or ignore it. This at least gives the child the chance to share feelings.

Parent: *Maybe you feel afraid there will be bullies at school, or maybe you're worried about being left out.*

Parents Can Use "I" Messages Instead of "You" Messages

- The "I" message allows parents to express themselves in a nonthreatening, nonjudgmental manner that makes the listener more open and more likely to accept the message.

For example, the following statements exemplify times when "I" messages should be used:
— *"I feel worried when you do your homework so fast."*
— *"I can't clean the house with all the toys out."*
— *"I feel angry when you swear."*

The "I" message communicates the effect of the child's behavior on the parent instead of suggesting that the child is inherently bad because of his or her behavior. When "I" messages are used, the child is more likely to assume responsibility for the behavior.

- Conversely, the "you" message sounds like a personal attack and conveys a put-down. The following are generic examples of "you" statements:
— *"You are just trying to get me mad."*
— *"You do your homework too fast."*
— *"You leave your toys out, and I can't clean up."*

The child often reacts defensively (with denial, resistance, anger, or ending the conversation) to "you" messages.

Parents Can Substitute "Yes" for "No" When Stating a Condition for Participating in Some Activity

"Yes" should be the first word the child hears when a parent attaches a condition to a child's request. Doing so acknowledges the child's need or desire and reduces conflict. For example, a child might say, *"Can we play ball?"* The parent's response should be, *"Yes, when you have finished your chores,"* instead of *"No, we can't because you have not finished your chores."*

Parents Can Explain Their Reason for Saying "No"

Children are more receptive to a "no" when the parent briefly explains the reason why. A parent can briefly elaborate by saying, *"We need to leave in 5 minutes to be on time,"* instead of *"No, you cannot play now."*

Parents Should Acknowledge the Child's Point of View

When parents acknowledge their child's point of view, the child feels validated because his or her feelings have been recognized (eg, *"I know it's hard to leave the party during the middle of it."*).

Parents and Children Can Learn to Apologize to One Another

Parents and children often say hurtful things to each other. Therefore, both parties need to be able to apologize by saying, "I'm sorry." Both also must be willing to forgive and to accept a sincere apology when it is offered. Effective communication may not be possible until the hurt feelings are addressed. For example, if a parent gets angry and says something hurtful, he or she should apologize to the child by saying, *"I'm sorry for hurting your feelings. I was angry. I didn't mean to do it."* If a child swears at a parent or says something insulting, the child likewise should be taught to apologize in a sincere manner. Parents need to teach children to say, "I'm sorry" when necessary. When parents say "I'm sorry," they should not expect or ask the child to forgive them right away. Hurt feelings take time to mend.

FAMILY RULES

Satir believed unspoken, unconscious rules of communication of families often inhibit self-expression. These rules, which determine what members can or cannot ask for, talk about, think, and feel, can put each member at risk for a variety of social and psychological problems (eg, inhibiting the expression of feelings and needs may lead to low self-esteem or externalizing behaviors such as acting out). Children unconsciously follow these rules, which are reinforced by disapproval, withdrawal of affection, or fear of punishment. For example, if the father becomes angry or disapproving when a child is fearful or needy, the child learns to repress those feelings. Children learn these rules and patterns from parents who learned them from their parents. Thus this style is passed on from generation to generation. Spouses often adopt each other's rules in order to maintain their relationship (eg, don't ask for emotional support). Some examples of family rules are listed in Box 20.1.

Box 20.1. Examples of Family Rules

- Don't ask for attention.
- Don't ask for help.
- Don't admit feelings of loneliness, sadness, hurt, or disappointment.
- Don't show anger toward parents and relatives or disagree openly.
- Don't seek positive feedback and praise for your work.
- Don't ask for emotional support or show affection.
- Don't talk about or ask about sexual feelings or orientation.
- Don't talk about your own or others' problems (eg, alcoholism, depression, abuse, affairs, hostility, or alienation in family relationships).
- Don't express uncertainty and doubt, especially within the family.

Case Study 20.1: Family Rules

First Child-Focused Visit

The father of a 10-year-old girl makes an appointment because his daughter Fran has been *"kicked off the school bus."*

The bus driver's report states that Fran suddenly pushed a girl off the seat. A fight ensued, after which Fran was warned and her parents were notified. The very next day, Fran threw a boy's backpack out the window. The result was that she lost bus privileges for a week. The parents are concerned about the behavior but also are very stressed because they now have to drive Fran to and from school, causing problems at work. Fran is generally *"quiet and well-behaved."* She earns good grades and has good health. The parents deny any recent stresses on Fran. Fran herself is cooperative, and her affect is appropriate. She cannot explain these fights, and the parents cannot understand her behavior. The clinician suggests that *"a few family discussions at home would help her talk things out."* He explains how to carry out home family meetings and schedules a follow-up visit in 2 weeks. (See Chapter 30.)

Second Child-Focused Visit

At the next visit, Fran's parents report that she has been ordered to sit by herself behind the driver on the bus, so she *"feels embarrassed."* Another problem has come up—the teacher suspects her of stealing her classmates' pencils. Fran denies it, but her parents have removed TV privileges for 2 weeks. The parents have not tried conducting home family meetings because they are *"too busy and tired"* in the evenings. The clinician speaks with the parents alone and then with Fran. He thinks that Fran might have an attention-deficit/hyperactivity disorder or a kind of behavioral impulsivity. He mentions conducting a more formal evaluation and the possibility of medication, but the parents are hesitant. The clinician suggests home family meetings again, saying *"I know you all have lots of feelings that a few good talks will help."*

Third Child-Focused Visit

A meeting is set for 2 weeks later, but the mother calls after 5 days. The teacher has reported that Fran is *"cheating on tests and is being isolated by friends."* The clinician, at a loss, feels that a family meeting is warranted. He explains the purpose to the mother, who agrees to it.

First Family-Focused Meeting

Understanding the Family

During the family meeting, the clinician first reviews the past interventions. The family has not used family talks because *"they don't feel right,"* but they are unable or unwilling to elaborate on the reason why. The family history is negative for medical or psychosocial problems. He again inquires about recent stresses, defining this as *"any change that affects the family."* The mother states that she and her husband are both busier with work and explains how that leaves less time and energy for home life. Also, a maternal aunt is going through a *"nasty divorce,"* so the mother visits or calls her frequently, which takes even more time away from the family. When asked why they hadn't revealed this in the first meeting, the mother replies, *"You just asked about Fran."*

The clinician, trying to understand the family's communication habits, asks if they have much time for conversation. The father responds with, *"We talk about work and home activities."* Watching TV is the major family activity. When he asks the parents if they talked to Fran about how she feels, they give him a quizzical look and say, *"Not really."*

The clinician asks about Fran being "isolated." With some gentle prodding, Fran begins to tell how she has been "pushed out" of her group of friends and that she doesn't know why. When the clinician asks her how she feels, she hesitates and then says, *"Mad and sad."* The parents had not heard about the problem with the friends until Fran mentioned it. They hadn't realized how upset Fran was. *"We didn't ask. I wish she had told us. We never know her feelings."* Therein lies the problem, the unspoken family rule: **No one asked. No one told.**

Fran's eyes fill with tears, and her body shakes with crying. The mother puts her on her lap.

Working With the Family

The clinician considers all the factors influencing the parenting practices, home life, and Fran's behavior. He knows that sharing his own "explanation" of the family dynamics to a family with unconscious rules would not be productive. But he does feel that he can share other information: The family is experiencing stress at work, the aunt's divorce drains the mother's energy and time and, as a result, the family has less time together. Fran has good reason to feel upset, but she hadn't told anyone. The clinician explains, *"Sometimes kids express their feelings with these behaviors."* He points out that Fran has many strengths, including loving and supportive parents, her health, and school learning.

During 3 meetings the clinician and the family develop some plans together.

1. The parents and the clinician agree to help Fran express herself—*"To help her do more talking and less fighting."* The focus is on Fran, which the parents are comfortable with.
2. The parents take turns arriving home about the same time as Fran does.
3. The mother tells Fran's aunt that she cannot see her as often.
4. The teacher is asked to investigate the problem between Fran and her friends but can find no obvious reasons for their behavior.
5. The teacher gives Fran extra help with her schoolwork, which eliminates Fran's cheating.

6. The stealing of pencils stops as Fran gets the attention she needs.
7. Fran finds another group of friends with the teacher's help.

As a result of these changes, Fran's behavior improves. The parents' communication style stays the same, but their efforts to modify their work schedule and home behaviors convey a feeling of love and support, and make a positive change in the family.

Family "rules" are unspoken and unconscious. The clinician should not challenge them or try to "explain" them unless the family seems open and receptive. The clinician can help the family in other ways, as this case illustrates.

Why Children Appear Not to Listen

Parents often complain that children "tune out," don't listen, or don't appear to listen. Children usually don't consciously decide to "tune out," but other explanations exist that clarify their difficulty in listening to their parents.

- Parents communicate at a level above the child's receptive language ability.
- Parents don't state their expectations clearly.

Clinicians can help parents appreciate their children's level of language development in many ways. Several milestones are listed in Table 20.1. Of course, normal variation must be considered, and the clinician and parents should remember that boys tend to develop speech and language more slowly than girls.

Case Study 20.2: Mother Talking Above the Child's Listening Ability

Well-Child Visit

A mother brings her 5-year-old daughter Lynn in for a regular well-child visit. As the visit is concluding, the mother lists several things she wants Lynn to do.

"Lynn, put on your shoes and get your book."

"Then we are going shopping and I expect you to behave."

"When we get home, you can help me with dinner."

Lynn suddenly turns to her and yells, *"I won't and you can't make me!"* The mother, embarrassed, takes Lynn by the arm, raises her voice and tells her, *"You do what I say!"* Lynn then begins to cry and throws herself on the floor. The clinician asks if this happens at home, and the mother replies, *"She yells at me whenever I ask her do something, and I would like some help."* The meeting is almost over. The clinician offers one suggestion: The mother should try to reduce her yelling at Lynn. The clinician schedules 2 family-focused visits and explains this to the mother.

Table 20.1. Expressive and Receptive Language Development		
Age	**Expressive Language**	**Receptive Language**
18–24 months "Terrific twos" tantrums begin	Knows 20–100 words; uses short sentences, 2 words ("Me cookie"), with 2 exchanges	Points to objects when pointed out; recognizes names of familiar people, objects, body parts; follows simple instructions
Age 2–3 years (greatest variation in this phase) Tantrums and mood swings common; is "selfish" and self-centered normally; little control over emotional and behavioral impulses; curious and active	Knows 200–300 words; uses 3-word sentences ("Where is doggie?"); says name, age, gender; recognizes most common objects; begins to express affection	Follows 2-sequence command; understands most simple sentences; understands concept of "2"; confuses reality and fantasy (may cause worry); beginning to understand "mine," "his," or "hers"
Age 3–4 years Views self as whole person: body, thoughts, feelings	Knows 300–1,000 words; uses 4-word sentences; begins to express thoughts and feelings; speaks clearly so that most is understood; begins to negotiate solutions to conflicts; "no" is a common word; responds to where, what, who	Can listen to and repeat grammatically correct sentences; listens to stories; recalls part of stories; follows 3-step simple command
Age 4–5 years	Knows 1,500 words, which will increase by another 1,000 by age 6; uses 5- to 6-word sentences; tells longer stories; can act/sound bossy (often repeating commands he or she has heard); may use swear words (often repeating what he or she has heard)	Recalls much of a story; can distinguish fantasy from reality; follows a 3- to 4-step simple command

First Family-Focused Visit

Understanding the Family

During the follow-up meeting, Lynn plays quietly with toys while the clinician takes a more detailed history. The mother is 25 and single, and the father has "disappeared." Her parents, who live in town, enjoy babysitting Lynn and are supportive. The mother drinks socially and denies drug use or affective problems. She is in good health and states that *"I love Lynn. She's all I have, but sometimes I just lose my temper with her."*

Lynn is in kindergarten all day and attends a child care program after school until 6:00 pm. Both mother and daughter come home tired. Shortly after arriving home, the mother usually begins issuing commands. The clinician asks the mother to recount an example of a communication problem with specifics about actual words that were used, the tone of voice, and the facial expression.

"Lynn, clean your room and when you finish, put your toys away, then wash your hands, and come help me in the kitchen, okay?" The mother's tone of voice and facial expression are stern, not friendly, and she expects Lynn to comply right away. When Lynn dawdles, the mother repeats the command in a louder voice and with a very stern look. Lynn's response is to yell back, so the mother threatens to spank her (which she never does) or to send her to her room (which she does).

The clinician recognizes 2 problems: The mother's talking exceeds Lynn's language abilities, and her general demeanor is negative so it hinders effective communication. These communication problems contribute to the disturbance in their relationship.

Working With the Family

The clinician asks Lynn, *"Do you want to say something?"* Lynn shakes her head. She gives Lynn paper and crayons and asks her to draw a picture of *"you and Mommy doing something."* While Lynn draws, the clinician explains the issues. She knows Lynn well and feels that she has a normal level of language development. The mother's commands are vague (*"Clean up your room."*) and overly long (4 sequences), and are delivered with a negative emotional intensity that discourages listening. Together, these factors overwhelm Lynn's abilities, so she responds in a negative emotional manner. The mother in turn responds emotionally, and soon they are both caught up in a problematic interactive pattern that often leaves them in tears. (See Chapter 26.)

The clinician asks the mother what she thinks she could do.

She replies, *"Talk with fewer sentences and sound friendly?"*

The clinician suggests that the mother make only 2 requests initially, using a maximum of 6 to 10 words and maintaining a neutral facial expression, while sitting at Lynn's level and making eye contact. The clinician discourages yelling and threats. Goals for Lynn are to make eye contact, listen, and follow her mother's directions. She's encouraged to ask her mother for a clarification or repetition.

Then she asks the mother and Lynn to role-play an interaction in the office.

When assigning a task or new behavior, the family should practice it in the office if feasible.

Mother (using the suggestions): *Lynn, look at me. Let's pretend it's bedtime. I need you to do two things. I will ask you just once. Change into your pajamas; then bring me your storybook.*

Clinician (to mother): *Now tell her to repeat what you said.*

The mother does.

Lynn: *Put on my PJs and get my bedtime book.*

Mother: *That's good. I like the way you listened and answered.*

The mother gives Lynn a hug.

Clinician (to both Lynn and her mother): *Can you do this at home?*

They both nod. The clinician reminds the mother that, at times, Lynn will make progress but progress is not always steady.

Second Family-Focused Visit

At the follow-up visit 2 weeks later, the mother reports that she and Lynn have had about a 20% success rate, which she feels is a definite improvement. They have 3 more visits over the next 2 months. At the last visit, the mother reports a 50% improvement. She is satisfied and feels she does not need to return.

Together, the clinician and the mother had developed some of the following strategies:

1. The mother understood Lynn's language abilities.
2. The mother adjusted her instructions to fit Lynn's abilities.
3. The mother adopted a positive demeanor.
4. The mother asked Lynn to make eye contact with her. She reminded Lynn to ask for repetitions and clarifications.
5. The mother rewarded Lynn for her effort and progress.
6. The mother arranged her schedule to have time for herself.
7. The mother would meet on a regular basis with a friend who also has a 5-year-old daughter.

Specific Issues and Solutions When Children Appear Not to Listen

- **Parents' communications exceed the child's short attention span.**
  - *Issue:* A child's optimal attention span is about 3 to 4 minutes per year of life (up to about 20 minutes), which is shorter than most parents realize.
  - *Solution:* The clinician should explain normal attention spans to the parents (eg, a 4-year-old child has an optimum attention span of 12–16 minutes in a calm and distraction-free environment and when engaged in a motivating task). But if the child is tired, anxious, or distracted, the attention span is greatly reduced. Therefore, the parent should reduce the time of sustained listening appropriately.

- **Parents talk over children's heads.**
  — *Issues*
    - Sometimes parents deliver too much information or speak too rapidly, exceeding the child's memory and processing abilities (eg, *"First, I want you to brush your teeth. Then lay out clothes for tomorrow and start your homework. Then finish your chores."*). The child may remember "finishing chores" but will remember nothing else.
    - Parents use "big words" that children can't understand because they surpass the child's developmental–cognitive ability (eg, use of "democracy" with a 5-year-old child).
  — *Solutions:* Parents can
    - Use smaller "chunks" of information (eg, 1, 2, or 3 short sentences).
    - Slow the rate down and speak slowly.
    - Use simple, familiar words that children have in their vocabulary.
- **Parents are not clear about what they want or expect from the child.**
  — *Issue:* Parents often issue commands that are too general and vague (eg, *"Be good,"* *"Behave,"* *"Do better,"* or *"Stop misbehaving."*).
  — *Solutions:* Parents can
    - State their expectations clearly (eg, *"I want you to do your homework. That means you must finish the ten math problems on page 23."*).
    - Pause and calmly ask the child if he or she understands what the parent expects (eg, *"Do you understand?"*).
    - Ask the child to repeat or paraphrase what the parent said (eg, *"Would you repeat what I said?"*).
    - Encourage the child to indicate if he or she needs clarification (eg, *"Mommy, I don't understand."*).
    - Use concrete, specific examples (eg, *"Remember how you cleaned up your room yesterday? You picked up the clothes, put them in a drawer, and then made your bed."*).
    - Demonstrate what is being asked of the child (eg, *"Let me show you how to do it first."* or *"Let's do it together first."*)
- **Parents expect children to respond quickly to a request, even if the child is involved in an activity.**
  — *Issues*
    - Parents do not give the child an advance warning that allows the child to finish one task and then prepare to listen to a request from the parent.
    - Children often feel that parents don't appreciate their needs to pursue their own activities and that sometimes they are not ready to respond suddenly to a parent.

— *Solutions:* Parents can

- Let the child finish a task, such as playing a game or watching a TV show, before making the request.
- Give the child a signal or warning (eg, *"In 3 minutes, we need to stop the game, and then we will speak."*).
- Adjust their schedule or priorities so that they fit better with that of the child's activities and interests (eg, *"I can wait until after dinner to discuss this."*).
- Set a convenient, regular time to converse with the child.

- **Parents' "emotional" message (eg, anger, frustration) often interferes with the child's understanding or willingness to respond to the verbal message.**
  - *Issue:* Anger, frustration, and irritability are "heard" first by children, and the other message (directive, request, explanation) is "lost" in the emotional message.
  - *Solutions:* Parents can
    - Self-monitor their emotions, body language, facial expression, and tone of voice (eg, *"I'm feeling pretty upset."*).
    - Step back, take a deep breath, count to 20, or take a time-out to calm down (eg, *"I need three minutes for myself before we talk."*).
    - Ask the spouse/partner (if available) to take over and/or to be primarily involved in a particular task (eg, directing the child to do homework or getting the child ready for bed).
    - Acknowledge the child's emotions (eg, *"I can tell that you are pretty upset about what I said."*).
    - Avoid humiliating the child (eg, *"Are you crying again?"*).
    - Apologize (eg, *"I'm sorry. I didn't mean to be so angry or hurt your feelings."*).
    - Teach children how to apologize.

- **Parents don't detect children's feelings or understand their thoughts and perspectives.**
  - *Issues*
    - Children feel that parents have forgotten what they (parents) were like when they were children.
    - Children may be worried or sad; they often express these feelings through behaviors that parents criticize. Their underlying feelings go unrecognized.
  - *Solutions:* Parents should
    - First try to understand the underlying cause of children's behavior before reacting to the behavior.
    - Remember and share a similar experience from their own childhood.

- **Parents' communication is often critical, judgmental, and hurtful.**
  - *Issue:* Children feel that parents don't notice what is right and that they focus only on what is wrong.
  - *Solutions:* Parents can
    - "Catch" their children doing something right. Recognize good behavior instead of just taking it for granted and ignoring it.
    - Give a new accomplishment, a good effort, or any small positive change the recognition, praise, and reinforcement that it deserves.
    - Record positive efforts and changes in a notebook and share them at a home family meeting.
    - Appreciate children's differences and respect their right to be different.
    - Ignore many inconsequential negative behaviors—often they will disappear. Parents must realize they can't attend to every negative behavior. They must "pick their battles." Parents also must focus on what's right, and what's working. Parents should "pick their victories."
- **Parents' communication often is too task-oriented and too directive.**
  - *Issues*
    - Children are always being told what, when, and how to do something.
    - The communication contains too little humor, affection, playing, or just being together with no specific agenda.
  - *Solutions:* Parents can
    - Provide unstructured time together. Just being together yields the possibility of enjoyable and unexpected things.
    - Find time to express affection and approval to their children.
- **Parents are often discussing their personal matters or problems in the child's presence.**
  - *Issue:* Children don't necessarily want to hear the details of their parents' personal problems. Children often become anxious or confused when they hear about adults' problems, especially when the children are treated as confidantes or are expected to provide support or advice. Children don't have the emotional or cognitive abilities to respond to their parents' needs.
  - *Solutions:* Parents can
    - Avoid exposing children to their personal problems in a way that makes them anxious.
    - Seek help for themselves from friends, relatives, and professionals.
    - Reassure children that they are seeking help for themselves.
    - Nourish and support their children's developmental needs as children. Children should not be "adultified" or "parentified."

- **Parents' communications are often repetitive and predictable.**
  - *Issue:* Children don't bother to listen. They "tune out" because they expect to be bored by their parents' communication. For example, a child might think *"It's the same old thing"* or *"Here comes lecture number 78"* when a certain subject comes up.
  - *Solutions:* Parents can
    - Monitor the content and repetition in their communication.
    - Surprise their children by saying something outrageous, funny, and unpredictable.
- **Commands and Requests**
  - Parents issue commands and make requests of their children. Sometimes parents make a request when they should make a command and vice versa. The following case illustrates these issues.

Case Study 20.3: A Tired Mother Slaps Her Son in the Office

Visit for a Camp Physical

A mother brings her 9-year-old son Jeremy to the clinician for a summer camp physical examination. The clinician notices that the mother is not her usual energetic, talkative self and instead looks quiet and worn out. After the examination, the mother tells Jeremy that he has to do some errands with her. Jeremy protests, stating that he wants to go the mall. The mother explains several times that they have other things to do, but every time he protests *"Why not?"* in a whiney voice. The mother clearly becomes exasperated, and when he yells, *"You're just an old bag!"* she slaps him. Jeremy begins to cry, and then the mother cries.

The clinician sits down with them both. He acknowledges their feelings and asks what is going on. The mother states that she has never slapped Jeremy before but that he always *"argues and makes me explain myself over and over. It's gotten so bad that I just let him do whatever he wants most of the time, but eventually I lose it. My husband tells me to be strict, but I can't; so things just get worse."*

The clinician tells the mother that he thinks a family meeting with her husband present would be very helpful and that he would like to schedule 2 meetings.

First Family-Focused Meeting

Engaging the Family

The clinician explains how the events of the past visit resulted in this meeting and that this family meeting is not just aimed at Jeremy. Its intention is to help all of them understand the problem and work together to resolve it.

The father says that she is *"too weak."* Jeremy pouts and refuses to answer. The clinician assures him that he is not being blamed and encourages him to speak up.

The clinician realizes that the mother's authority has been eroded because of the father's criticism of her. Therefore, the mother–child hierarchy has been altered, and the father needs to support the mother.

Understanding the Family

Jeremy sits by his father and away from his mother. The clinician wonders if a father–son coalition exists and works against the mother to undermine her authority. The father feels his wife needs to be more *"strict."* When Jeremy hears this, he states, *"I can always get my way."* He is proud of his ability to *"win arguments."*

The clinician decides to explore a specific problematic situation to better understand the family. The PCP asks the family to describe in detail a family challenge.

The mother replies that getting Jeremy to do homework is predictably difficult. When he gets home from school, he speeds off to watch TV, which is a daily source of conflict.

As Jeremy continues to watch TV, the mother asks in a polite manner, *"Jeremy would you turn off the TV and start your homework? Okay?"*

Jeremy, without taking his eyes from the TV, answers, *"No, not now. Later, I promise."* He also states a few reasons why he needs to relax and rest before doing his homework.

The mother returns to the kitchen, comes back in 20 minutes, and makes the same request. This time Jeremy usually answers that he doesn't need to do homework now because, *"I can do it all in 20 minutes."* Again he gives his mother several reasons why he doesn't really need to do the homework now. The mother then requests that he show her his homework assignments. Again Jeremy explains that he will show it to her later. Then the mother asks Jeremy if he would like her help with his homework. When he refuses her offer, she loses her temper and tells him that she will have his father speak with him when he comes home. Lately however, she has *"given up because it's easier than arguing."*

The clinician realizes that the mother's repeated requests give Jeremy several options for getting his way: ignore, refuse, procrastinate, and argue. Eventually, he will wear his mother down. The clinician asks the family members what they would like to achieve. The mother's goal is to have Jeremy do what she asks. Together the clinician and the parents agree on this realistic goal. When Jeremy understands that there might be more *"peace"* in the family, he agrees. The boy needs a clear, firm command, not a polite request followed by much persuasion. Their communication pattern is not working for the mother and disrupts the mother–son relationship.

Working With the Family

The clinician asks the father what he means by *"strict."* The father explains that it means *"giving orders when you have to."* This is a command. The clinician asks him to demonstrate. The father faces his son at eye level. He puts his face about 12 inches from his son, assumes a stern expression, and orders in a slow, deliberate manner, *"Jeremy, I want you to turn off the TV, go right to your room, and start your homework. Do it **now**."*

The mother asks Jeremy if that would make him obey her. With a somewhat startled expression on his face, he says that it would. The mother says that she could make such a command but that she needs the father's support, and she asks him to *"back me up, but don't criticize me."* He agrees to help out. With his support, she becomes more confident and uses commands, not requests with Jeremy. Jeremy responds positively. There is indeed more "peace" in the family.

Below are other examples of communication breakdowns.

- **Interrupted commands**
  - *Issue:* The parent continues talking beyond the initial command or makes irrelevant requests, which confuse, distract, and delay the child. For example, a mother might say, *"Please go and clean up your room and then do your math homework. Before you do that, help me put away these dishes.* Interruption: *Remember the last time I asked you to clean your room? You really argued with me. I hope that doesn't happen again."*
  - *Solutions:* Parents can
    - Keep the message short and simple and focused on the major request.
    - Make a mental note to wait to introduce other topics until after the first task has been completed.
- **"Let's" requests**
  - *Issue:* The "let's" requests may imply a lack of parental authority or parent–child differentiation in situations when differentiation is appropriate (eg, *"Let's go clean up your room."*).
  - *Solutions:* Parents can
    - Change the request to a command.
    - Make the requests so that they are perceived by the child as a way to spend time with a parent and to gain the parent's approval. This then provides a chance for the parent and child to cooperate and to share. In this way, the parent is modeling good behavior. For example, the parent might say, *"Let's work in the garden together. I bet that you could really help me. We'll have lemonade after we finish."*

- Avoid making the requests and then either not joining in or leaving before the task is completed. Then the requests become a form of deceit or disappointment. If the parent has been doing this, then the parent should either stop using requests or should work with the child until either the task is done or they both agree to quit.

- **Repeated commands**
  - *Issue:* Excessive repetition allows the child to figure out the parent's maximum number of commands or "boiling point," at which time the parent "explodes." The child "tunes out" until just before that "boiling point" is reached. Then the child finally "listens" to the parent and complies.
  - *Solutions:* Parents can
    - Understand that the child has figured out the parent's limit.
    - Use the 1-2-3 rule. With the 1-2-3 rule, the parent explains to the child that he or she will only request or command 3 times in 15-second intervals and specifies the consequences for both obeying and disobeying. Then the parent gives a command in an appropriate manner (calm, firm voice, eye contact, short command) and says, *"That's one."* The parent looks at the child, waits 15 seconds, and repeats the command with *"That's two."* He or she should wait another 15 seconds and repeat, if necessary, with *"That's three."* After another 15 seconds, the parent should act according to the consequences he or she laid out. If the child complies, a suitable positive reinforcement should follow; if the child doesn't comply, an appropriate negative consequence should be immediately applied (eg, time-out or a restriction of a favorite activity). Corporal punishment is discouraged.

- **"Nattering"**
  - *Issue:* The parent repeats commands, the child ignores them and, ultimately, the parent gives in and does the task himself or herself, muttering, *"It's easier to do it myself rather than to tell him to do it 6 times."*
  - *Solutions:* The parent can
    - Understand how his or her behavior maintains the problem.
    - Prioritize what is most important (eg, the parent "picks her battles" or "her victories").
    - Allow the child to experience the logical consequences of his or her actions (eg, *"If dirty clothes are not put in the hamper, soon you will have no clean clothes to wear."*).

- **Requests and questions that imply equal power**
  - *Issue:* The parent asks a question or makes a request in a way that implies equal power (eg, *"Wouldn't you like to go to bed now?"*). This gives the child the opportunity to refuse, bargain, or manipulate.

— *Solutions:* Parents can

- Change their request to a command (eg, *"I want you to come over here **now!**"*) to convey a sense of proper parental authority.
- Offer 2 acceptable alternatives or choices. *"You have a choice to set the table or clear the table. Which one do you choose?"*
- Recognize and reinforce the behavior with a kiss, hug, or smile.

- **Threats.** The use of threats often causes the family to focus more on the threats developing than on desirable behaviors. Threats cause resentment, anxiety, and sadness; and they put pressure on the parent to carry them out. Additionally, to remain effective, threats often have to increase in severity, creating a potentially dangerous environment for the child. Moreover, if threats are not carried out, they lose their coercive power. So, in the end, threats are not effective.

  — *Issues:* Described here are several different types of threats.

  - The parent combines a threat and a command. These commands evoke confusion and tension and possibly even negative emotions or actions, such as anger, refusal, regression, hurt, fear, resentment, or guilt. *"I want you to finish your homework and be in bed by nine o'clock. If you don't do it, I'm really going to spank you."*
  - The parent may threaten to hurt himself or herself. (eg, *"I'm going to go crazy!"* or *"If you don't do what I say, I'm going to kill myself."*)
  - The threat made by the parent is disproportional for the misdeed (eg, *"No TV for a month"*), or it can imply physical harm (eg, *"I am going to whip you."*).
  - The parent may threaten to abandon the child, saying something like *"I'm going to walk out this door and never come back."*
  - The parent's threat may damage the child's sense of self-worth and ability to feel loved. The parent may say, *"Sometimes, I wonder why I had you,"* or *"I wonder why you turned out so bad."*

  — *Solutions:* Parents can

  - Understand that empty threats are ineffective and may instill fear and anxiety, and that real threats to harm a child may lead parents to be overly punitive or violent. Parents should never
    - Threaten to hurt themselves because of the child's behavior
    - Threaten to abandon the child

    To develop empathy in the parents, the clinician might ask the parents to imagine they are the child and to imagine how the child might feel. Also exploring "parenting history" may reveal that the parents themselves were disciplined this way.

INVALIDATION BY FAMILY MEMBERS

Invalidating communication patterns diminish one's sense of self-worth and discourage communication between family members. Ways in which communication patterns invalidate a family member are described below.

- **Generalizing statements**
  - *Issues*
    - Generalizing statements imply that a child can never do any good. Examples include, *"You're always disobeying me"* or *"You never take responsibility for anything."* If the parent has these attitudes, then the child will always feel like he or she is a disappointment to the parent and can never measure up. This engenders in the child a sense of shame and failure.
    - Whenever something goes wrong, the child is always blamed. For example, if the child brings home a poor school grade, the parent assumes the child is at fault and blames him or her without first investigating. He or she may say to the child, *"There you go again— more lousy grades. What's wrong with you?"*
  - *Solutions:* Parents can
    - Stop using generalizing terms like "always" or "never" in a negative way.
    - Seek to understand first before judging or assuming.
    - Learn that comparisons between siblings may cause the child to feel that he or she does not measure up. Rather than compare, parents should help each child develop his or her unique skills and interests. The child can't do this alone.

- **Evading statements or actions**
  - *Issues*
    - Parents find ways to evade a discussion or avoid a meeting/interaction with the child. The parent can pretend not to hear, respond with silence, or postpone the conversation. For example, a father might say, *"Ask your mother," "I know you want to talk about the baseball game, but I am too tired right now,"* or *"Wait until this weekend."* Eventually, the child begins to feel unwelcome and unimportant and stops approaching the parent.
    - A parent can avoid a child by being unavailable either physically or emotionally, such as leaving home early, coming home late, retreating to the bedroom, sitting in front of the computer or television, or appearing harried and unapproachable.
  - *Solutions:* Parents can
    - Respond to the child's needs at the moment.
    - Put off some of their activities until the child is busy with homework or in bed.

- Set aside "special time" on selected evenings for activities and conversations. (See Chapter 30)

- **Disqualifying statements**
  - *Issue:* The parent praises the child in a qualified manner. *"Congratulations on the B you earned in math! I am proud of you. But if you'd only studied like I said to, you could have made an A."* The result of such qualification is that the child feels that he or she can't ever do enough to please the parent and that he or she is a loser, not a winner.
  - *Solutions:* Parents can
    - Encourage the child and help him or her make a renewed effort.
    - Recognize and reward the effort and/or success; let the child savor it.
    - Appreciate the developmental level of the child and set new, appropriate expectations and goals.
    - Ask the child his or her own opinion of the grade.

- **Closing a discussion prematurely by way of verbal and nonverbal messages**
  - *Issues*
    - Verbal messages, such as, *"I have to go,"* *"I don't have time to listen to this,"* and *"You make me so mad I'm leaving"* make the child feel unimportant and disrespected.
    - Nonverbal messages, such as rolling the eyes in disbelief, averting them from the child's gaze, turning one's back on the child, standing up, glaring at the child, yawning with feigned boredom, walking away, looking at TV, or reading the paper, discourage communication.
  - *Solutions:* Parents can
    - Put aside their activities for the time being.
    - Permit the child to conclude the conversation.
    - Set another time to talk, if necessary.
    - Ask questions and show interest.

- **Unwanted advice**
  - *Issue:* Parents often offer advice or suggestions when the child does not want it or is not ready for it. Examples include, *"Let me tell you what you ought to do,"* *"Listen to me,"* or *"When I was your age, I did...."*
  - *Solutions:* Parents can
    - Hear the emotional message behind the verbal message.
    - Determine if the child might only be seeking praise and support but not advice.
    - Tell the child that the parent is always available if the child wants advice.

- **Guilt trips**
  - *Issue:* Guilt trips happen when one family member tries to get attention by inducing guilt, often by letting others know that he or she is in pain or by using sad facial expressions, sighs, and stories of past pain. Making

children feel they are disappointed induces guilt in children. The message, either verbal or nonverbal is, *"If you cared for me you would stay home"* or *"After all I do for you, you treat me like this."* Eventually others tire of this behavior, become exasperated, and pull away.

— *Solutions:* Parents and the family can discuss methods of helping the person using guilt trips so that they meet his or her needs in other ways. When parents use guilt trips, children become sad, resentful, and avoid the parent. If the clinician detects this in a family meeting, he or she should first speak to the parent privately and respectfully.

INEFFECTIVE COMMUNICATION PATTERNS

Ineffective communication issues involve various family members. Members are often unaware of these patterns and of their own contributions to them. Types of ineffective communication patterns and solutions for remedying them include the following:

- **Denial**
  - *Issues*
    - Denial occurs when a family member does not want to recognize another's feelings or need to communicate. Examples of denial statements are *"I don't care,"* *"No problem,"* *"Whatever you say,"* *"It doesn't matter,"* or *"You don't really feel that way."* Associated behaviors might be slouching, shrugging, withdrawing, speaking in a monotone voice, or avoiding eye contact.
    - Stonewalling is a form of denial. Stonewallers are silent, unresponsive, and unrevealing. They often withhold love and approval and don't readily expose their own thoughts and feelings. Stonewalling affects children deeply and causes pain, self-doubt, anxiety, and distrust. Stonewallers confuse children because they don't know what to expect from the stonewaller and they don't get needed feedback. A stonewaller doesn't allow children the chance to interact; therefore they don't feel loved or validated.
  - *Solutions:* The clinician can
    - Help the family understand its behaviors and how it affects individual family members.
    - Help the family members acknowledge the feelings of others in the family meeting.
    - Take the parenting history. The PCP asks each parent how each of them was parented. How did their parents communicate, express affection and disapproval, or spend time with them? It is sometimes best to excuse a child when taking a parenting history.

- **Indirect expression**
  - *Issue:* Indirect expression means a veiled way of stating one's needs or desires. The speaker does not plainly express himself or herself, so the listener does not hear the real message. For example, a family member might say, *"It's been quiet around here"* instead of *"I am lonely and would like you here."* Or the child might say, *"Boy, this homework is hard"* instead of *"I need some help and encouragement."*
  - *Solution:* The clinician should help the family members express their needs with a direct statement that starts with "I." Members can become more perceptive, sensitive, and responsive to other's expressions of need.
- **Substitutions**
  - *Issue:* Substitutions allow an expression of feeling in a safe way or with a safer person. For example, a father who is angry with his wife instead may get angry with his son; or a parent who feels hurt or neglected when a teenager stays in her room all the time criticizes her friends or the quality of her schoolwork instead of telling her he feels neglected. Another example is an older sister who can't express her secret happiness about her brother's success at school so she worries about his eating habits instead.
  - *Solutions:* The clinician can
    - Help the family express what they want and need in a clear, calm manner (eg, *"I would like..."* or *"I am feeling...."*).
    - Help the family listen to and acknowledge the feelings and thoughts of others (eg, *"I hear what you're saying,"* or *"I sense you are feeling...."*).

Chapter 21

Salvador Minuchin: The Structural Family Model

*T*he Minuchin model is based on modifying the organization of the
family with a view toward the present and future, not toward the past.
The focus is on the family system or structure, the invisible (but powerful)
functional demands/expectations/obligations that define roles and organize
how family members interact.

SYSTEMS

The family is a system or organization that functions through repeated
interactional behaviors that determine how, when, and with whom members
interact and relate. The pediatric care professional (PCP) "joins" the family
system and helps the family members make changes that might be helpful
(eg, changing hierarchy relationships and roles, thus changing the structure
and functioning). The family has a hierarchy, a power structure, or an order of
those with authority or rank. The PCP must determine "who is in charge" and
be sure to form a good relationship or alliance with the "family CEO." Power
struggles may also exist within the family. Roles are the assigned expectations or tasks, spoken or unspoken, often defined by ranking in the hierarchy.
Minuchin states several principles.

- Man is not an isolate, does not exist alone.
- A family member's psychological and emotional life is not entirely an
  internal process.
- The family structure influences the behavior and inner-psychic life of
  each member. Changes in the structure generate new behaviors and
  psychic processes.

- The behavior of the PCP, when working with the family, becomes part of the family context. The PCP joins with the family to help it form a new, healthier, better functioning system that then governs the behaviors of family members.

Subsystems

Family systems consist of subsystems that may be 1 person (eg, a son or a parent), 2 persons (eg, husband and wife, brother and sister), 3 persons (eg, a mother and 2 children or 2 parents and 1 child), or more persons. Subsystems in turn are separated and distinguished by boundaries, a collection of rules (spoken and unspoken) that dictate who participates and how in a particular subsystem. For example, the marital and parental subsystems define the participants and their power, roles, and behavior.

Subsystems are in constant motion; they interact with and change other subsystems. Changes may occur within a subsystem; for example, a parent may become ill or the parents may divorce. So the parent subsystem is changed, which affects the spouse–partner and the sibling subsystems.

Families generally have 3 subsystems. Each requires well-defined boundaries.

- The parents' subsystem gives the child access to both parents or partners (or to 1 parent if single) while limiting access to the spouse or partner domains. Raising and socializing a child is naturally challenging, and an intact parent subsystem maintains the appropriate parent–child hierarchy and functions.
- The spouse–partner subsystem requires a boundary to protect it from intrusions and demands by the other subsystems, specifically the children. This subsystem provides a refuge for the adults' own emotional, sexual, and intellectual needs and for support for each other.
- The sibling subsystem allows children to develop their relationships: cooperation, competition, sharing, problem-solving, empathy, protectiveness, role-modeling, and individuation. These skills are employed and further developed outside the family with other peer relationships.

HIERARCHY

Hierarchy is the power structure that defines leadership and authority. Who is in charge (eg, the parents, the child, a grandparent)? How does he or she assert authority or get his or her own way? Families are not democracies. Parents normally are in charge, but sometimes inappropriate hierarchies exist so that the children control parents. Other determinants of authority include age (eg, an older sibling is in charge of younger ones) and gender. Mothers tend to be in charge of family function, emotional well-being, and day-to-day parenting responsibilities. Fathers tend to be major providers and ultimate authority figures and may take some responsibility for daily family–parenting roles. However, these traditional roles are changing.

Within the family system, subsystems comprised of 1, 2, 3, or more persons exist. The major subsystems, which are the marital/partner, parental, and sibling groups, all affect each other. Therefore, when a clinician encounters a parent–child issue, he or she should also inquire about other subsystems that influence the problem and/or that are influenced by the problem. Roles are often "assigned" to subsystems and/or to specific members in the subsystem. The roles are intended to carry out the family's tasks. For example, nurturing and socialization are the roles of the parental subsystem.

BOUNDARIES

Boundaries are 2-way streets of interaction with easy access or limitations and emotional closeness or distance. They specify who enters or stays outside of a subsystem and determine how members should interact. They provide guidelines for privacy, intimacy, and communication as well as rules for how family members interact with and relate to one another. Boundaries provide the rules and expectations that protect subsystems. They must be clear to all family members and yet flexible enough to allow contact between subsystems. For instance, the spousal and parental subsystems are "protected" from the sibling subsystem by clear boundaries. Most importantly, boundaries define emotional relationships (eg, appropriate, too close, or too distant). The spectrum of boundary clarity ranges from enmeshed (overly close and too engaged) to disengaged (distant, estranged); clear and appropriate boundaries exist in the middle of that continuum. However, all families at different stages of the family life cycle experience these 2 extremes temporarily (eg, a parent may be enmeshed with an ill child or a teenager may be disengaged from the family). In families with behavioral and interaction problems, the clinician finds that boundaries are often blurred, confusing, and problematic. Three types of boundaries and relationships are described below.

1. **Diffuse boundaries.** Diffuse boundaries appear unclear, limit individual autonomy, and provide little private space. They result in enmeshment where family members become over-involved in each other's activities and personal lives. Anyone can enter another's subsystem (eg, the parents— marital/partner subsystem—have no privacy or time for intimacy; a child continuously interrupts his parents' conversation or telephone calls). A mother and son are enmeshed when the mother answers all questions for her son at any age or wishes to be present when the clinician performs a physical examination on a teenager. When enmeshment occurs, family members rarely act independently. The family is too emotionally reactive; thus any level of stress causes an immediate family response.

2. **Rigid boundaries.** Rigid boundaries, those that are unyielding and inflexible, allow very little contact or interaction between subsystems. The family system is characterized by disengagement, and the members are emotionally distant, withdrawn, and unresponsive to each other (eg, a father rules by firm, authoritarian means and appears unapproachable; a child is experiencing emotional stress at school but does not tell her parents). The family resists change. These disengaged families lack family cohesion and mutual support, and children receive little individualized attention and guidance. When rigid boundaries exist, families require a high level of stress to activate a supportive family response.

3. **Clear boundaries.** Clear boundaries are appropriate and apparent between subsystems (eg, the marital subsystem and the children). Each subsystem remains functional and healthy and maintains contact with other subsystems. Relationships allow communication and cooperation within the appropriate hierarchy—the parents are in charge.

The PCP uses knowledge of the system, subsystems, hierarchies, and boundaries to understand the family structure and function/dysfunction, which in turn generates and orients therapeutic interventions and suggestions to change the stressed systems; eliminate maladaptive, repetitive behaviors and interactions; change alignments; and allow for constructive problem-solving. The mission of the PCP is to facilitate changes in the family system by joining the family in a position of "leadership"; evaluating and explaining the underlying "dysfunctional" family structure and creating circumstances or offering suggestions that allow change of the structure. The PCP enters this encounter knowing that he or she is primarily responsible for what happens.

Chapter 22

Jay Haley: The Problem-Solving Model

*I*n the Haley model, the focus is on solving the family's presenting prob-lem. The pediatric care professional (PCP) helps define the presenting concern and constructs an intervention within the family's social situation. This model emphasizes the social context of family problems and the family's adaptability. The PCP must develop the ability to give directives or suggest tasks successfully.

- Directives or suggestions help families behave differently.
- Directives or suggestions may be used to strengthen a relationship between the family and the PCP.
- Directives or suggestions are used to gather information. A family reveals itself according to how it responds. Every therapeutic attempt is also a diagnostic probe.

Directives or suggestions fall into several categories.

- Telling the family members what and when to do something
- Telling a member to stop doing something
- Telling a member to do something different, whether intended for an individual or a directive to change the member's sequence of behaviors in the family

Giving good advice assumes that the family is rational and has control; however, sometimes "good advice" does not work if the family is not ready for it, or if the advice does not "fit" their beliefs or level of coping. In that case, the PCP assumes responsibility for that "failure" and considers the next step. This problem-solving method assumes that family members interact in pre-dictable, repetitive sequences based on the family's organizational behavioral pattern. The PCP determines the sequence and attempts to change it. For this to be successful, parents must be motivated and in agreement. Directives should be specific, realistic, meaningful, and achievable. The best directives involve all family members, with each member having a specific role.

The PCP should feel free to selectively take specific aspects of various models and combine them into a workable model that fits him or her and the family situation. For example, the PCP may combine aspects of the Satir, Minuchin, and Haley models, as illustrated in the following case study in Chapter 23.

The Family With a Son With Attention-Deficit/Hyperactivity Disorder: Selected Examples of the Satir, Minuchin, and Haley Models

CASE STUDY 23.1: THE PHONE CALL FROM THE PARENT

The mother of a 14-year-old boy (Bobby) called because he *"won't take his medication after school."* The clinician knew Bobby but really did not know the family well. He had diagnosed Bobby with attention-deficit/hyperactivity disorder (ADHD) and was treating him with stimulant medication. The school had provided accommodations for his attention problems. The clinician remembered the boy as being well-adjusted both socially and emotionally. The mother added that *"his behavior is concerning all of us."*

Clinician (determining who is involved, who is affected): *Who do you mean by "all of us?"*

Mother: *All of us. Me, my husband, Bobby, and his brother, Randy. Everyone is stressed out. We don't know what to do.*

After a few more minutes of conversation in which the mother kept referring to the stress on the family, the clinician suggested a family meeting.

Clinician: *I'd like to suggest that we have a few family meetings. That means I'd like your husband and Randy to come in too.*

The clinician scheduled 3 meetings. Before the first meeting, he reviewed Bobby's chart.

First Family Meeting

Engaging the Family

1. **Greeting the family.** The clinician greets the family and asks the family members to seat themselves as they wish in a semicircular pattern. He notices that Bobby uses this opportunity to distance himself from his parents.
2. **Social conversation.** Previously, the clinician had not met the father. He converses with him for a few minutes to establish an alliance with him. He hasn't seen Randy (17-year-old brother) for a year and inquires about how he is doing. He speaks with the mother and Bobby.
3. **Stating the purpose of the family meeting.** The clinician wants to be sure that everyone is clear about the purpose of the meeting and is in agreement. He addresses each member, not just the mother, and does his best to make sure that Bobby does not feel like he is "the problem."

Clinician: *Let's be sure we all agree on why we are meeting. We're here because you all want to resolve a challenge that is affecting the whole family. Bobby, this means you alone are not "the problem." Everyone is involved and everyone will help. Would anyone like to comment?* (alternatively, *"Is this right?"* or *"Do you agree?"*)

Mother: *The problem is that Bobby has ADHD and won't take his after-school medication.*

The clinician scans the other members for their responses.

Father: *Whatever she says is right.*

Identifying the Leader

The clinician identifies the mother as the family leader.

Bobby (adamantly disagreeing): *That's not right! I'm here because they made me come.*

Bobby is the "identified patient" and the clinician wants to acknowledge his feelings.

Clinician: *"I appreciate you being here. I realize you didn't want to attend the meeting."*

The clinician wants the family to understand the purposes of the meeting and the shifts in focus (a) from the adolescent–patient to the family context and (b) from parents "reporting" the issue to the clinician to a family conversation with all involved.

Clinician (again clarifying the purpose of the family meeting): *I want to point out that these family meetings are to help all of you understand that the concern is really a family issue. No one person is to blame, and no one person has to do all the work. Everyone is affected, but together as a family you are the best resource for solving this issue.*

By the looks on the family member's faces, the clinician can tell that all of the family members seem a little surprised by this statement.

Clinician (permitting 10–15 seconds of silence as they considered his explanation): *You seem a little surprised. What do you think is the purpose of our meeting? What would you like to see happen in our meeting?*

One by one, he asks each member; each nods—they are surprised, but the purpose becomes clear. The purpose is to resolve the family issue about Bobby, his mother, and the medication. **The family must understand the purpose and agree on it before the clinician can proceed.**

Avoiding Coalitions

If the clinician had agreed with the mother and father, the family might perceive his action as forming a coalition with the parents against Bobby. By taking sides and acting like another parent, he would certainly have lost Bobby's trust and cooperation.

Clinician (giving Bobby a chance to respond): *Is there something you'd like to discuss at this meeting?*

Bobby (revealing he wants to change his place in the hierarchy, an aspect of the Minuchin model): *They treat me like a baby. I'm doing fine. I don't need it.*

Clinician (acknowledging Bobby): *Just what do you think you need or want? You have the opportunity now to share your thoughts and to speak your mind.*

Bobby: *To have them get off my back about the meds.*

Clinician (to parents): *What do you think about this?*

Parents: *We just want to end this arguing.*

Clinician (getting Randy involved): *Randy, what do you want?*

Randy: *It seems like the medication thing is a stress in our house. They're always yelling about it.*

Clinician (instilling some hope): *The fact that you all are here, sitting in one place and willing to talk, means that you have taken the first step to improving things.* (The pediatric care professional [PCP] attempts to see if the family can agree to this shared strength as a starting point for a goal discussion.) *It sounds like the decision about whether or not to take the medication is the issue that is causing so much stress in the family. Is that right?*

He asks each member to answer. One by one they agree.

Managing the Family's Expectations for the First Visit

To ease the family's urgency to "get to the bottom of this" in one meeting and to relieve pressure on the clinician to "fix the problem," the clinician should tell the family early in the first visit that a first visit is meant to gather information and understand the family, the concern, and their goal. Later in the first visit, or in the second visit, the PCP will help the family develop ways to work together and possibly offer advice.

Understanding the Family and Their Concern

Families usually expect to talk about the concern, and the clinician needs to understand the concern within the family context.

Clinician (encouraging everyone to participate and using the word "concern" more than "problem" because it carries less stigmatization): *I'd like to hear more about the concern from all of you.* (This implies a certain amount of "equality" among each member. It allows Bobby to define a less-enmeshed relationship with his mother and to establish a new role.)

Mother (talking to the clinician): *He just refuses to take his medication and to study at home, and I end up nagging him because high school grades are so important for college.*

Clinician (discouraging the mother from "reporting" to the clinician about Bobby and encouraging family communication): *Look at Bobby and tell him how you feel.*

The mother voices her concerns to Bobby.

Clinician (continuing to promote family communication): *Bobby, would you like to say anything?*

Bobby: *I feel upset too.*

The clinician looks at the father and Randy to offer them the opportunity to respond. They both look glum and nod.

Clinician (acknowledging the family's mutual feelings): *It seems like everyone is upset.* (To the father who has been quiet so far) *How do you see things? Would you add your thoughts?*

Father: *When Bobby arrives home after school he wants to "hang out," but I know he will not study in the evening. His mother tells him to take his medication and study. He won't take his medication. That starts a big argument between them. That's the problem.*

Clinician (gently challenging the father's statement): *How do you know he won't study in the evening?*

Father: *I assume he can't without medication.*

Bobby (looking at the clinician): *They think I need my medication all the time and that I can't do anything on my own. I can study better after dinner when*

I've had a chance to relax, play some music, and talk to my friends. I'm doing fine in school, but they don't believe me.

Practicing a Desired Behavior in the Office

If the clinician wants to improve family communication, he must facilitate effective family communication in the meeting. If they cannot carry out a constructive conversation about the desired behavior (goal) in the office, they probably will not be able or willing to do it at home. This reflects an aspect of the Satir model.

Clinician (promoting family communication): *Bobby, tell your parents, not me.*

Bobby: *Mom, I can do my work better after dinner. Just give me a chance to show you. I am doing fine in school.*

Mother: *We haven't seen a report card yet.*

Assessing Behaviors That Maintain the Problem and Its Impact on the Family

Clinician: *How has this issue affected the family?*

Father: *Sometimes Bobby skips the family dinner.*

Bobby: *I'd come downstairs to dinner if Mom didn't always get so intense.*

Mother (looking at the clinician): *I worry about Bobby. I'm always checking up on him.*

Clinician (again encouraging family communication as in the Satir model): *Does Bobby know how you feel? Tell him how you feel.*

The mother looks at Bobby and tells him. Bobby meets her gaze but remains silent.

Clinician: *Have you told Bobby what you worry about?*

Mother: *No.*

Clinician: *Do you want to now?*

Mother: *Not right now.*

Randy: *I don't even want to come home and face their arguing. I hang out with my friends.*

Mother (her eyes filling with tears): *I've tried so hard.*

The clinician pauses and allows 10 to 20 seconds of silence. He waits for a family member to break the silence. No one does, so he speaks.

Clinician: *It must be hard for you. You seem saddened by this situation.*

The mother nods quietly. The father reaches out and holds her hand. Bobby looks away, still angry. Randy looks at his parents.

Clinician: *Tell me how you've responded to this issue.*

Mother: *We're not really working together. We are all so busy with other things.* (This is a cue for some advice in the Haley model.)

Father: *We don't really have a plan. It's kind of chaotic. Every day I just hope things will get better, but they don't. The yelling just keeps getting louder.*

Randy: *Like I said, I just hang out with my friends. I don't know what to do.*

Mother (still hoping the clinician will "fix" Bobby's "problem"): *We're here for you to talk some sense into Bobby.*

The clinician avoids playing the parent role. He does not give advice at this time. The family is not ready. He has not yet gained the trust of the family. He repeats that this is a family issue.

Clinician (guiding the family): *Remember, I am not the expert. You all are. You have the answers. Bobby, we promised you'd have an opportunity to speak. Let's hear from you.*

Bobby (still angry): *I don't want to be treated like a baby. I told you that.*

Mother (still looking to the clinician for advice): *But you are the expert. That's why we're here.* (The mother has not yet tried to construct her own solution.)

Clinician (maintaining the family systems approach): *I can help, but this meeting is to help you all become experts.* (This puts the family back in the driver's seat.)

Identifying Family Changes That Affect the Problem

Clinician: *Were there any other things going on about the time the problem began?*

Father: *I was under pressure at work. I put in longer hours.*

Mother: *We never see each other. We don't have a moment together.*

When parents express or hint at a need to feel supported as parents or spouses, the clinician should simply acknowledge their need, even briefly, but should not get distracted and ignore their presenting concern. The clinician can also discuss other issues later on in the meeting or in the next meeting.

Clinician: *That must be hard.*

Father: *We haven't gone out in months.*

Mother: *We're too worried.*

Clinician (noting the mother has twice mentioned being worried): *You've mentioned your worrying a couple of times. Now can you tell Bobby what worries you? Look at him and tell him.* (This is enhancing communication as in the Satir model.)

Mother: *I worry that you won't study, won't get good grades, won't get into college, won't get a good job, and won't have a good life, like you have now.*

Bobby (softening a bit): *Mom, you're worrying about everything. You tell me what to do all the time and even remind me to brush my teeth.* (Bobby is trying to assert his independence and place in the hierarchy.)

The family is silent.

The clinician feels that the mother is overly involved with Bobby, is micromanaging his activities, and is stressing the family in the process. The boundary is too diffuse.

Clinician (identifying adolescence as a challenge in the family life cycle, and reminding them of a past success): *I remember when Randy was Bobby's age. We had a talk about his need to separate and become an individual. He wanted a little more independence. You gave him some room, and he did fine.*

Mother: *But Bobby has ADHD. Randy didn't.*

Bobby looks hurt.

The clinician considers the idea that the mother feels Bobby's ADHD makes him vulnerable. Does this make her overly involved in his activities? Cause her worry?

Clinician (probing gently): *Do you think that Bobby needs more supervision because of his ADHD?*

The parents look at each other and nod.

Clinician (to Bobby): *How does that sound?*

Bobby (looking a bit less tense): *If Mom gave me a chance like she did Randy, she'd see that I can do it too.*

The clinician also wants to acknowledge this normal phase/stress of the family life cycle.

Clinician: *Bobby is going through the same stage of adolescence as Randy did, and he has the same developmental needs to separate and be independent. It can be a stressful transition for families each time it happens.*

Father: *It sure is.*

Discussing Past Attempts and Advice to Resolve the Problem

Clinician (seeking useful school information): *As there is a focus on medication and studying, it would help to get some information from the school and to know what they might be doing to help Bobby. I will give you a teacher questionnaire, and you can bring it to our next meeting. What have you tried in the past?* (This is an example of the Haley model. The PCP may also review how ADHD was initially diagnosed.)

Bobby: *I did try medication in the afternoon, but I just wasn't ready to study then and it took away my appetite for dinner.*

Clinician: *Anything else?*

Bobby: *My parents had me see the school counselor a couple of times. He was okay. He told me I was doing fine.*

Father: *I used to help Bobby with homework after dinner. That worked for a few weeks, but then demands of my job stopped that.*

Clinician (acknowledging a past success): *So something did work, even if for just a while.*

Father (remembering his own success): *I suppose.*

Clinician (exploring other attempts and advice): *Has anyone offered you any advice?*

Mother: *A friend of mine who has a boy the same age as Bobby said I should find something else to do in the afternoon instead of nagging Bobby. I haven't done it.*

Clinician (exploring their readiness for advice): *Would you like to try?*

Mother: *I'm not sure.*

Clinician (keeping Randy involved, and helping him get the respect he wants): *Randy, do you want to add something?*

Randy: *Nope.*

Discussing a Goal

A brief goal discussion helps the family clarify its expectations. It is also an effective way to end a problem discussion that has gone on too long, become repetitive, and/or turned the interview into an angry blaming session. Goal discussion precedes advice giving.

Clinician (shifting the interview focus from the problem to a goal): *We've talked about your concern. Now I'd like to ask each of you what you'd like to achieve in these meetings. If this issue were gone, what would you want instead?* (Recognizing Bobby's need for autonomy and separation.) *Let's hear from you first, Bobby.*

Bobby: *I want to have afternoons free and to study at night.*

Randy: *I want things to be easier at home.*

Father: *I just want Bobby and his mother to settle down.*

Clinician (seeking clarification): *Can you both be a little more specific?*

The father and Randy mention having a pleasant dinner, maybe watching TV after dinner, and letting each member have time alone.

Mother: *My goal is for Bobby to take his medication and study.*

Clinician (attempting to get agreement on a goal by showing how the goals are all connected): *It sounds like you all want pretty much the same thing... that is to have pleasant evenings and have your own time. Working out this medication–study issue is kind of a step toward the goals. I'd like to offer a suggestion. Tell me what you think. How about Bobby doing homework with* *and without medication? Then you all can discuss the results.* (The clinician now exerts some leadership by offering a general suggestion.) *Bobby could study at night without medication and show that he can do well. Once we see what works, we'll know what will help the family get along. How does this sound? If it is not successful, he could take medication in the afternoon and study then.*

The family nods in agreement. Bobby and his mother both appear a bit relaxed for the first time in the visit.

In the short office visit, this is a good point to end the first meeting.

Concluding the First Meeting

The conclusion should summarize the meeting in a positive way that emphasizes the family's effort and achievements.

Clinician: *In this first meeting, we talked about your concern as a family issue and you all talked about it, and then we discussed your goal. Resolving the medication issue and study time will make family life more pleasant. It seems like you want the same goal. There are things going on that affect everyone, like Dad's job changes, Mom and Dad not having time for themselves, and 2 teenagers who are going through adolescence. It's obvious you care for each other and are willing to work together on this goal. I've proposed a solution (inviting the family to ask questions or share thoughts). I'd like to hear any final thoughts or questions.*

The clinician allows a period of silence to let the family gather its thoughts.

Mother: *What do we do now?*

Clinician (encouraging the family to try something on its own and avoiding the expert–parent role): *What would you like to do?*

Father (taking the lead): *Maybe Bobby and his mother can compromise. I like the suggestion that he take his medication after school for three days and study before dinner, then not take his medication for three days and study after dinner. Then we can talk to Bobby, compare the homework, and decide on the best plan.*

Mother: *For the sake of peace, I will try it.*

Bobby (reluctantly): *Just this week.*

Families sometimes modify a suggestion so they are all satisfied.

In this case, the clinician feels the father's suggested strategy will work. It is the father's idea and he hopes it will help the mother and Bobby to change their behaviors. The mother and Bobby have not discussed this goal in detail, which may be for the best, as it might avoid another argument. The clinician supports the father, who is obviously trying to assert some family leadership. Time has run out, so he makes no objection. The clinician compliments the family for its willingness to try this strategy.

Scheduling the Next Meeting

Clinician: *I'd like to schedule our next meeting in one week. Can you all attend?*

Clinician (complimenting and thanking the family): *I want to tell you how impressed I am with your commitment to each other and your willingness to join together in this strategy.* (Pauses for a few moments to let the positive message sink in.) *In our next visit, we will discuss how your plan worked out. We might discuss other ways for you to work together. Work on your plan this week. You've made good progress. Please call me anytime with any questions or concerns. Thank you for coming in.*

Post-Interview Phase (First Visit)

After the family leaves, the clinician reviews the first meeting. He feels that the family is satisfied with the family meeting and is willing to come back. He is pleased with how he conducted the meeting, and he likes the family. He realizes that much of the conflict originates from the mother's perception that Bobby can't work without medication and that he needs to study in the afternoon. The mother seems very worried that Bobby's "untreated" ADHD will cause him to underachieve. She projects her worries into the future and worries that he won't have a "good life." Bobby needs and wants more autonomy. The parents need to be assured that Bobby can behave responsibly. The family wants more harmony. Several issues need attention: family patterns of interactions; beliefs about Bobby, ADHD, and the developmental needs of adolescents; and inadequate time for the parents' own spousal life. The clinician determines that he will help the family prioritize the issues and address them over the next few meetings.

Second Family Meeting

The PCP can tell immediately by the family members' facial expressions that they aren't pleased. They look disappointed and avoid eye contact with each other as though they have "failed." The clinician inquires about the past week. The compromise worked for only 2 days. The father reports that Bobby wanted all his afternoons medication-free, so the arguments started again.

Clinician (acknowledging their feelings): *I am sorry things didn't work out. I sense you might be feeling a bit discouraged. Let's hear from each of you.*

The clinician looks at each member. Everyone is silent.

Clinician (reminding them of a strength and that they aren't failures, keeping them hopeful): *Last week you showed a family strength. You were willing to compromise and try something new. Even though it didn't work out, let's begin with these strengths.*

Sometimes starting with positives when the family is feeling discouraged is much more helpful than rehashing the problem at the risk of making them feel even worse or having the members start "blaming the patient" again. Using the phrase "didn't work out" is better than "failed."

Working With the Family

Identifying Family Strengths and Resources

Clinician (to the father, reminding him of a past success): *At our last visit you mentioned that you used to help Bobby with his homework and that it was helpful.*

The father and Bobby agree that it was.

The clinician asks for the teacher questionnaire in the hope that he might find a strength/success at school. He quickly glances at it. It does suggest Bobby has ADHD, but it also contains some very positive comments.

Clinician (to both parents, exploring Bobby's strengths as a way to demonstrate his capabilities and to elicit an indirect compliment): *He does have mild ADHD. At the last visit, I mentioned we'd also explore some of Bobby's strengths. Have you shared these comments with Bobby?*

The parents had picked up the form on the way to the meeting and had just glanced at it in the waiting room. The clinician asks them to share the comments with Bobby. They read them. Bobby is doing grade-level work and is well-behaved. Bobby's ADHD is mild, especially when he has a structured learning environment. The teacher suggests Bobby may be *"maturing out of his ADHD."*

Clinician: *How does that make you all feel?*

The parents state that they are *"a bit surprised"* and *"very pleased."*

Clinician: *Would you tell Bobby?*

The parents look at Bobby and compliment him.

Clinician: *How does that make you feel, Bobby?*

Bobby (smiling): *Proud.*

Clinician (exploring other strengths): *Bobby, what else do you do that makes you proud?*

Bobby states that he has a part-time job and that he had just gotten a raise, which brings more praise from the clinician and the parents.

Clinician (complimenting the parents): *You've done a good job of being parents. Look at how well Bobby and Randy are doing. Can you give Bobby a chance to show you how responsible he is?*

Father: *I'm willing. It seems that with maturity and success, his ADHD is diminishing, and he is more capable. We need to let him show us.*

Mother: *How can we do that?*

Engaging the Family in a Plan of Action

The clinician decides to answer the mother's question by pointing out the father's support.

Clinician (reviving a past success to create a plan): *Bobby has said that he can study at night and that Dad's support was very helpful. Could that happen again?*

Bobby nods, and the father states that he can help out when he comes home early.

Changing Roles

Mother (still doubtful): *I'm not sure about this. My husband could help maybe one night. That leaves me doing most of the supervision. That's not really a change.*

One of the most effective ways for families to change their interactions is to change roles. One member "steps out" of an interaction, and another "steps in." In this family, the mother will not give up her role of supervising Bobby unless someone else steps in. She is not yet ready to give Bobby the amount of independence he wants and needs. She still feels he needs supervision and medication. Bobby wants to feel trusted and responsible.

Father: *I could be home earlier two or three nights per week.*

Clinician (facilitating discussion on how help the mother "let go"): *Remember, Bobby has shown that he is responsible. Who else could we find?*

Mother: *Maybe a tutor?*

Father: *They are expensive.*

Clinician (scanning the family, hoping Randy might "step in"): *It is a family effort. Does anyone have another suggestion?*

Randy (responding to the "family effort"): *Maybe I could help out a couple days a week. If things are calmer at home, I wouldn't mind coming home.*

This offer represents a significant change in the family's pattern of behavior. The clinician wants to emphasize that Randy himself would benefit from this effort.

Clinician (complimenting Randy): *That's really generous of you. So you get to enjoy a calm house and wouldn't have to stay away. How does that sound to all of you?*

Bobby: *I'd like that.*

They all agree that it's worth a try. The mother asks the father and Randy *"to set a schedule now, so there would be no slipups."* They do that in the office.

Clinician (to all): *Well done.*

Offering Advice (Haley Model)

Although the family has developed a plan, the presenting complaint (from the family leader) has not yet been addressed. The mother will not be satisfied until her specific concerns are addressed.

Clinician: *Have we settled the after-school medication issue?*

Mother: *Shouldn't he take medication after dinner?*

Bobby: *I tried it once and it kept me awake.*

Clinician (offering a specific directive): *Bobby, how about this? When you have a lot of studying or a test, it might help to take the medication an hour before dinner. That would help you, and it shouldn't interfere with your appetite or sleep.*

The family now realizes this addresses both the medication and moving the homework time. It changes family roles and changes behaviors and perceptions. This gives Bobby a chance to be more responsible.

Bobby (indicating his willingness to take medication after the positive family discussion): *I could try it.*

Clinician (offering more advice): *Sometimes, studying with a classmate can be helpful. Bobby, do you have a friend who you could study with if Randy and Dad can't make it?*

Bobby: *I could study with Mel. He's a good friend and a good student. We could try that.*

Mother (still wanting to help, to be involved, to have some control): *I could help out with the driving.*

Clinician (recalling the parents' concern that as spouses they had little time for each other): *Maybe now you could find some time for yourselves. The boys are doing well. Go out on a date. You deserve some fun too.*

Both parents: *That would be nice.*

Clinician (complimenting the family): *Look how much you all have accomplished. Everyone was heard and you have agreed on a plan that satisfies everyone.*

Changing Perceptions and Providing Reassurance

The clinician quickly reviews the psychosocial need of adolescents to be more autonomous. He reminds the parents of the boys' individual strengths and once again lists the teachers' positive comments about Bobby: His ADHD is well-managed and he is doing well in school. He gently urges the mother to focus on the next few weeks instead of the next year. Finally, he also reminds the parents that they had trusted Randy with more independence when he was Bobby's age. Could they do that with Bobby?

Assigning Homework Tasks (Optional)

Sometimes the family benefits from a task that makes it "practice" its new behaviors. The task emphasizes the desired behaviors and each member's specific roles. The purpose of the task is to have them record and remember the family successes.

In this case the clinician doesn't want the family members to "forget" the changes or to take each other's improved behavior for granted.

Clinician: *I'd like to assign the family a homework task. How does that sound?*

Mother: *Will it take lots of work?*

Clinician: *Some work.*

Bobby: *Is it like schoolwork?*

Clinician (laughing good naturedly and helping them relax): *Nope, and it will help you all remember the good things you've worked on here.*

Mother: *Tell us what you have in mind.*

Clinician: *I'd like you to get a notebook and call it "Good things I see and do."* *Put it in the kitchen or family room. Whenever anyone does something good or when you see someone doing something good, write it in the notebook. Share the notebook together every week. Do you think you can do that?*

Randy: *Maybe we'll mention the pleasant dinners we haven't had for a while.*

Concluding the Second Meeting

Clinician (pausing and then looking at each member to signal the conclusion): *I'd like to take a moment just to summarize all you have done today. Your concern was the afternoon homework, Bobby's medication, and the family stress. You agreed on a goal and together developed some specific solutions: Dad and Randy working with Bobby, using a study buddy, Mom doing the driving, and the family carrying out the plan that Dad suggested. The family cooperation is very impressive.*

The clinician pauses for 10 seconds to let the family reflect on his words and to consider any responses the members might have.

Clinician: *What comments or questions do you have?*

The parents say that they feel better. Bobby and Randy nod in agreement.

Clinician: *You've made some great strides. These were good visits. Congratulations to you all. Thank you for coming in. I'd like to see you all for a short visit in three weeks. Please call if I can be of any help before our next appointment.*

Post-Interview Phase (Second Visit)

The clinician reviews the meeting. He feels that the family is caring and competent. The members appear willing to change their behaviors. The mother's perception of Bobby has improved. He has helped the family in several ways.

- He clarified the purpose of the meeting and used a family discussion to resolve the problem.
- He encouraged the family to find its own solutions with a family approach.
  — The father offered to help out again.
  — The mother's perception of Bobby and his ADHD became more positive, and this changed her behavior. She "backed off," trusted Bobby and, in effect, trusted her own good parenting.
  — The clinician reminded the parents of Bobby's needs as an adolescent.
  — The clinician helped them change the family roles in the homework situation with both the father and Randy agreeing to help Bobby.
  — The mother offered to drive Bobby to his study buddy's house, thus removing herself from the homework situation.
  — The clinician supported the spousal relationship.
- The clinician offered advice/teaching/reassurance.
  — He suggested the notebook task.
  — He supported Bobby's choice to study in the evening and to take his medication before dinner, when needed.

Chapter 24

The Brief Solution-Oriented Model

*T*he solution-oriented interview differs from the problem-oriented interview because it focuses less on problem description and more on solution building. It shifts the focus of the interview to solution talk to shorten the problem talk and assumes that repeating preexisting successful behavioral patterns is easier than stopping or changing existing problematic behaviors. It views past and present strengths and successes of the family as the basis for future solutions.

Solution-oriented interviewing avoids generic ways of viewing and diagnosing family problems and generic therapeutic approaches ("one size fits all"), which often unintentionally deny creative possibilities to the clinician and the family.

Solution-oriented interviewing encourages co-constructing solutions, with both the family and the clinician viewed as "experts." The clinician conveys his or her need to know more about the family instead of merely testing preconceived values and notions. In this way, the clinician receives constant information about the family's values, traditions, and explanations so that he or she can better understand the family.

SOLUTION-ORIENTED QUESTIONS

The clinician then continues with selected questions that emphasize strengths, possibilities, and solutions. Problem-oriented questions, which can perpetuate discouragement, should be kept brief and asked at the beginning of the interview. Three solution-oriented techniques described below include goal discussion, exception questions, and scaling questions. The clinician should choose the one(s) that best seems to fit the family.

The solution-oriented interview is useful in the following situations:
- It allows families to make realistic, incremental changes.
- Problem talk is counterproductive.
- Families want solutions that fit their individual and cultural values.
- The clinician has a good relationship with the family already. This is a critical step to a successful outcome.

Goal Discussion

Goal discussion creates an atmosphere of hope, energy, and action that moves the family from the past into the present and future. The family engages in a discussion, which is often hopeful and optimistic, of what it wants to achieve. Several ways to initiate a goal discussion are listed in Box 24.1. Because families are usually unfamiliar with the solution-oriented questions, introducing them as "another kind of question" often helps.

Box 24.1. Ways to Initiate a Goal Discussion

- "What would you like to see happen as a result of coming here?"
- "Pretend you could fast-forward a video of your life 6 months into the future. What would you see?"
- "Imagine you woke up one morning and things were better. What would you first notice?"
- "What would tell you, after a few visits, that you wouldn't need to come here anymore?"
- Two questions for younger or less verbal children
  - "Wave this magic wand and make a wish. What would it be?"
  - "Pretend you have a magic crystal ball. Look into it and make believe that something good happened. What would you see?"

If the family still hasn't defined the goal as a positive, specific behavior that the members want to see more of, the clinician needs to help them do that.

Qualities of Well-Formed Goals

Families' goals, which are often too vague, are usually stated as desires for less of or absence of undesirable behaviors instead of as a hope for certain desirable behaviors. Clinicians must help the family state its goals as specific, positive behaviors that members can visualize. Qualities of well-formed goals include the following:
- **The goal is meaningful and important to the family.** The goal must arise from the family's frame of reference and its own value system.

- **The goal is realistic and achievable.** The goal should be small rather than large because achievement is more likely, which gives the family a sense of satisfaction and a feeling that the work is worthwhile. The clinician can provide an appropriate developmental perspective on the child (ie, goals that are appropriate for the child's abilities).
- **The goal has contextual, situational features.** The goal is a behavior that occurs in familiar, daily, or near daily situations (eg, doing chores, doing homework, obeying parents, playing with siblings, demonstrating affection, and communicating).
- **The goal is described in specific, concrete, behavioral, and interactional terms.** Observable, specific behaviors are more likely to be recognized and achieved. Families usually need guided discussion to attain this. A general goal like *"be good"* is vague and subjective; in contrast, a specific goal is, *"When I ask you to put your toys away, I would like you to put them in the toy box within 2 minutes."*
- **The goal is described as a positive observable behavior or the start of something new.** The absence, the ending, or the lessening of a negative behavior is not a goal; for example, *"I want no more fighting," "I want this arguing to end,"* or *"There will be less swearing in this house."* These examples are not adequate goals because they do not define or specify the desirable behaviors that would replace undesirable behavior. Families often have a hard time stating goals as positive behaviors because they have become so accustomed to discussing the problems and because they perceive the clinician as the problem-solver. The clinician can ask "exception-to-the-problem questions." *"What do you want to see happen instead of 'less swearing'?"* or *"What would happen if there were 'no more fighting'?"*
- **Families must perceive that achieving goals requires commitment and real work.** The clinician must tell the family that goals will be achieved only if the family is committed and willing to work. He or she must keep the family's expectations at a realistic level and should caution it with the reminder that disappointments or setbacks occur. Families usually improve their behaviors for a short time after each meeting because they are motivated to work on the behaviors. However, they often revert to their old ways because they don't remember or practice; they forget that achieving their goals requires consistent motivation and work.

EXCEPTION QUESTIONS

Exception questions shift the focus of the interview from problem talk to solution talk. This initiates a search for past successes. Exceptions are those behaviors that have occurred in place of the problem behaviors. By asking about them, the clinician aims to elicit what is working, what is going right, and what has worked in the past that the family might try again. They often also reveal goals. The clinician can ask exception questions instead of or in addition to goal questions, or with scaling questions.

Examples of these types of questions follow:

- *"If things were better, what would be different?" "What would be happening instead?"*
- *"Surely there must have been times when things were a little different. Tell us about one of those times."*
- *"When the problem is not happening, what's happening instead?"*

The purpose of exception questions is to reveal those times when the problem does not happen, is not so bad, is corrected, or is unnoticed. Their function is to uncover, identify, and explore those behaviors, feelings, thoughts, and perceptions that are exceptions to the problem because exception behaviors are the family's own real-life solutions. Therefore, discussing exception questions is the pathway from problem talk to solution talk.

SCALING QUESTIONS

Scaling questions serve 3 purposes: (1) they encourage each family member to "rate" his or her own sense of competence and hopefulness, (2) they help each member develop or improve behaviors and problem-solving strategies that move the family toward its goal, and (3) they promote family communication and cooperation because the family members respond to each member's "rating" and know they need to work together to achieve their goal. Overall scaling questions lead to family discussions, self-awareness, increasing their sense of competency, and defining productive behaviors. The clinician may use scaling questions alone or with goal or exception questions.

Children especially like the scaling questions because they are like playing a game. The clinician might ask children these questions first so they won't be influenced by the parents' replies. If the child cannot grasp the concept or is uncooperative, the parent should go first.

The clinician uses the following process to ask these questions:

- He or she says, *"I'm going to begin our meeting with a different kind of question. Sean, on a scale of 1 to 10, 1 represents the worst things have been and 10 is the best things could be. Where are you right now?"*
- The clinician always uses the answer to initiate a search for strengths. *"So you are at 4. That's pretty good. Almost halfway there. You must be doing something right. Tell me what you are doing to be there."* Or *"Ms Bowman, how has Sean gotten to a 4?"*

Everyone should participate so that a sense of cooperation, competence, and support is built. To emphasize the interactive context of family behaviors, the clinician then asks another relevant family member, eg, the mother, *"Ms Bowman, how have you helped Sean get to a 4?"* and *"Sean, how has your mother helped you get to a 4?"*

- In order to develop Sean's sense of responsibility, the clinician could ask, *"Sean, what can you do to get yourself to a 5?"*

This series of questions should also be asked of the parents. For example, *"Ms Bowman, where are you on a scale of 1 to 10?"* If she answers with a "4," then the clinician should ask *"Ms Bowman, what can you do to get to a 5?"* or *"Ms Bowman, how can Sean help you get to a 5?"* Examples of scaling questions are listed in Box 24.2.

Box 24.2. Scaling Questions

Assessing the problem
"On a scale of 1 to 10, with 1 being the worst the problem has been and 10 being the best things could be (if the problem were solved), how would you rate things right now?"

Measuring feelings
"On a scale of 1 to 10, with 1 being how you felt (happy, hopeful, sad, angry) when we first met 2 months ago and 10 being how you'd feel when you wouldn't need to come here anymore, how are you feeling now?"

Describing one's change in behavior
"So you went from a 5 to a 6. How did you do that? What did you do?"

Developing a new behavior
"You said you are at a 4. What would you need to do to go from a 4 to a 5? How would you do it?"

Describing interactive patterns of behavior
"How would Mom know that you have gone from a 4 to a 5?"
"What could you do to help your son go from a 7 to an 8?"
"How would your mother act when she sees you at an 8?"

Describing interactive emotions
"How do you think you would feel when your mother is at a 6?"
"How would your sister feel when you share your toys with her (when you're at a 7)?"
"How would you know she felt happier? What would you notice?"

The solution-oriented interview follows the same sequence as other interviews.

Box 24.3 lists the steps and questions of the solution-oriented interview.

Box 24.3. The Solution-Oriented Interview: Steps and Questions

1. **Engaging the family** (time: 3–5 minutes)[a]
   Social conversation
   Explain the purpose of a *family* meeting.
2. **Understanding the family** (time: 7–10 minutes)[a]
   Brief problem description
   Parenting history (optional)
   Behaviors that maintain the problem
3. **Working with the family** (time: 5–10 minutes)[a]
   Three questions (1 or 2 may suffice)
   - Goal discussion
   - Exception-to-the-problem questions
   - Scaling questions
4. **Concluding the meeting** (time: 3–5 minutes)[a]
   Summarize the meeting.
   Invite the family to ask questions or share thoughts.
   Schedule a follow-up visit.
   Compliment and thank the family.

---

[a]These times are approximations based on the number of questions and complexity of the case.

Chapter 25

An Example of the Solution-Oriented Model

CASE STUDY 25.1: A 10-YEAR-OLD BOY WHO "ACTS RUDELY ALL THE TIME"

The mother calls the clinician, stating, *"My husband asked me to call you for an appointment. Our boy is acting rudely, and we can't stop it."*

The clinician inquires about past interventions (family-initiated or professional). The parents have tried to be "stricter," but that has failed. They have not sought professional help.

The mother says, *"We come from a culture that says families should take care of their own problems. We have tried everything we know, but now we need help. As our son's pediatrician, we thought you could help."*

The pediatrician makes an appointment for a family meeting.

Engaging the Family

Social Conversation

The clinician hasn't seen Ricky and his mother in a year. She has not met the father until now. She starts the session by stating that it is good to see both Ricky and the mother again and that she is happy to meet the father. She notes that Ricky sits closer to his mother and looks worried. He doesn't smile and keeps glancing sideways at his parents. The clinician asks the father about his job, and she asks Ricky about school and other activities. Ricky pauses, and the mother answers for him, stating that he is doing well in school and has a lot of friends.

Clinician (deliberately writing this good news on his notepad and complimenting Ricky): *Well done, Ricky!*

Father (angrily): *But that's not the whole story.*

Clinician (acknowledging his anger and need to talk): *I see this is upsetting, I'll let you share your thoughts in just a moment.*

Explaining the Purpose of the Family Meeting

Clinician: *First, let me explain what I would like us to accomplish in this visit. This meeting is different from what happens when you bring a child in with a medical problem. Instead of focusing just on Ricky, we can address your concerns best by understanding the concern and the whole family together. As a family, you are an invaluable source of knowledge; and you have many strengths and resources. I'd like to learn more about both Ricky and the family so that we can develop solutions that fit your values. How does that sound to you?*

Father: *But I need to tell you about Ricky's bad behavior.*

Clinician (easing the pressure to do it all in one visit and adding a positive "spin" to the concern): *You will. That's where we'll start. First, we will briefly discuss your concern and see if you all agree on it. Then we'll discuss your goal and other issues that may affect the problem. Finally, I'll help you all develop some solutions. If we can't do all of this today, we will schedule another meeting. Then we'll have a few more visits after that. I know you and Ricky have some family strengths. I need to hear about those too.*

Father (speaking for the family): *I thought we only had this one visit. That makes me feel better. It's too much for one visit.*

The offer to schedule another meeting to complete the interview takes pressure off both the family and the clinician.

Understanding the Family

The clinician has reviewed Ricky's chart. He is healthy, and his immunizations are up to date. The only prior visits have been for well-child care and minor acute illnesses. She has noted that both parents were born and raised in Cambodia. They married there and came to the United States about 12 years ago.

Understanding the Hierarchy

Clinician: *Whose idea was it to bring Ricky in?*

Father: *Mine. In my country, we handle these problems at home. Or we get advice from relatives. We don't have relatives here. I've tried a few things, but the problem is getting worse. I told my wife to call you.*

The clinician identifies the father as the leader.

Brief Problem Description

The problem description should be brief.

Clinician: *Now I'd like to ask each of you to describe very briefly your concern.*
Father: *He acts rudely all the time.*

Clinician: *Can you give us an example?*

Father: *When he is at the table, he talks loudly and often in a disrespectful manner.*

Mother: *Ricky wants to talk and talk. My husband likes a quiet dinner. He tells him to be quiet. Ricky doesn't listen and keeps talking, raising his voice, and acting rudely. Then my husband yells at him to stop or tells him to leave the table. The dinner ends on a bad note.*

Father (angrily): *He's a rude child.*

Clinician (reframing the issue): *It seems like the talking at the table is the rude issue.*

Ricky: *I just like to talk.*

Father (angrily): *Loudly and nonstop.*

Clinician: *How long has this been happening?*

Mother: *It has been going on for several months.*

The clinician notes the father's negative comments and angry mood. She asks the mother how she responds. The mother replies that she does nothing. The clinician wants to end the nonproductive problem talk and also to stop the father's negative, angry comments.

Clinician (signaling the end of the problem discussion): *Is there anything else you'd like to add?*

Father: *We're tired of talking and yelling. Nothing gets better. That's why we're here.*

Clinician (acknowledging that they may need to "revisit" the concern): *If we need to discuss the issue again, we can do so. This information was helpful.*

Parenting History (Optional)

Clinician (exploring influences in the parents' behavior and expectations): *Sometimes it helps to know how you* (the mother and father) *were parented and how you were raised. For example, what were family meals like? How did your parents expect you to behave? Were there certain rules?*

The mother's parents had encouraged conversation at the table and insisted that everyone participate but would not allow them to interrupt one another.

The father's family dinners were *"very quiet."* His father was *"very strict."* He explained that in Cambodia, the father is the leader of the family and expects complete obedience. His father had been a *"traditional Cambodian father."*

The clinician senses that the father's childhood experiences are influencing his own parenting behavior. His rigidity and the rigid boundary may be part of the problem.

Father: *We had a rule that you only spoke when spoken to. If you broke the rule, you were sent to your room.*

The clinician attempts to point out the connection to the father between his father's style and his own style. If the father makes this connection, he might develop some empathy for Ricky.

The mother explains that she was raised by "more progressive" parents.

Clinician (to the father): *Did you enjoy the family dinners?*

Father: *Not especially. Dinner was the only time we were together, but I didn't get enough attention from my father.*

Clinician (following up on the father's own feelings): *Do you think Ricky is seeking your attention?*

Father: *Yes, but there are better ways to do it.*

The father has offered the possibility of a solution with this statement. The clinician responds to this "offer."

Clinician: *What are those ways?*

Father: *We're not sure. Nothing seems to work. That's why we're here* (again stressing his frustration).

Goal Discussion

The clinician feels that she is still missing something. She doesn't understand the family interactions as well as she needs to, so she needs more information.

Behaviors That Maintain the Problem

Clinician: *I'd like to hear an example of a specific incident at the table. I'd like to hear from all of you.*

The father states that Ricky will start talking about something that happened at school. After a few minutes the father asks him to stop. Ricky stops only momentarily and then will continue. The father again asks him to stop. Ricky persists. Soon the father and Ricky are both speaking loudly. The father then either raises his voice, which silences Ricky, or sends him to his room.

Mother: *Just like his father did to him.*

Clinician (seeking confirmation from the father and developing empathy for Ricky): *Is that right?*

Father: *Yes. I don't like doing it, but it seems to work.*

Clinician: *But the problem is still there. Does this happen a lot?*

Mother: *Over and over. I don't interfere because I do not want to disagree with him in front of Ricky. I get upset with him in private later, but it doesn't change things.*

Clinician (to Ricky): *What would you like to say?*

Ricky: *I hate it when Daddy sends me to my room.*

The clinician points out that the family is repeating the same behaviors over and over with increasing intensity. All of the family members are affected. The interactions have worsened despite their efforts.

She feels that this is a good point to shift to a goal discussion.

Clinician (introducing a new goal question): *Now I'd like to ask another kind of question. What would you like to achieve with these meetings?*

Father: *I want the rude behavior to stop.*

Mother: *No more unhappy meals.*

Ricky: *I don't understand.*

Clinician (asking Ricky to state a positive goal, using an exception question emphasizing the operative word "instead"): *You wished for no more yelling. What would be happening instead if there was no more yelling?*

Ricky: *Talking.*

Clinician (eliciting a more specific goal): *Tell Mom and Dad what you mean by talking.*

Ricky: *Just talking about school and things.*

The clinician wants to encourage a family conversation, a family interaction that the members could practice and continue at home. She asks them to role-play an interaction. (See Chapter 28.)

Clinician: *Pretend you are at home. I'd like you to have a family conversation. Would you tell each other what you'd like to see happening if there were "no more unhappy meals"?*

Mother (to Ricky): *Hearing your goal helps me understand things better. I would like to hear more about your school day.* (To the father) *I'd like it if you would let Ricky talk more. He wants to talk to you.*

Clinician (to the father): *Can you tell Ricky what you mean by "wanting the rude behavior to stop"?*

Father (to Ricky): *I'd like you to be quiet when I ask you.*

Clinician (helping them negotiate a goal): *It sounds like you all pretty much want the same thing—a pleasant, polite family conversation. How could you make that happen? Tell each other.*

Father (to Ricky): *I suppose I could let you talk more without raising my voice. I do like to hear about your school activities.*

Clinician: *Can you be more specific when you say "have quiet conversation"?*

Mother: *We could let Ricky talk first. He and I could begin a conversation, and my husband could join in if he wanted to.*

Clinician (to mother): *Would you look at Ricky and say that again?*

The mother's voice and expression soften as she speaks to Ricky.

Father: *I would like Ricky to be quiet when I ask him.*

Clinician (attempting to have family members talk to each other, and not to the pediatric care professional): *Tell Ricky that.*

The father does. Ricky looks at him but doesn't respond.

Clinician (bringing out the interactive aspect of behavior): *How could you help make that happen?*

Mother: *If Ricky had some time to talk and share his day, I think he could then obey his dad when asked.*

Father (in a softer voice and with a pleasant expression): *What do you think, son?*

Ricky (looking back and forth between mother and father): *I'll try.*

Clinician (helping them understand Ricky's behavior): *What else do you think Ricky wants?*

Mother (looking at her husband): *Our attention, especially his dad's.*

Father (remembering what he missed from his childhood dinners): *Like I wanted.*

Giving a Family Hope and Motivation

A brief problem discussion and a detailed goal discussion may constitute one meeting. More talk about where the family wants to go (goal) and less about where it has been (problem) leaves the family members feeling hopeful and motivated.

Purpose of Goal Discussion and Questions

The goal discussion and the exception and scaling questions help the clinician to understand the family and its goal and to work with the family. It is not necessary to ask all 3 types of questions. One or two will suffice.

Exception Questions

Clinician: *Tell me about a recent dinner when things were just a little bit better. What was happening instead?*

Father (after a long pause): *A few weeks ago, Ricky and I talked about a pro football game we had watched on TV.*

Clinician (acknowledging an exception and asking the family to elaborate on this positive behavior): *So you do have pleasant family conversations. Tell us more.*

The father and Ricky describe their behavior in more detail.

Clinician (looking for more exceptions): *What else has helped?*

Mother: *Last week, I asked Ricky to help fix dinner. As we worked, he told me all about school. At dinner, he didn't feel the need to talk as much.*

Clinician (pointing out their successes): *You've described two family behaviors that help you all have a pleasant dinner: when Ricky and his father talk about sports and when Ricky talks with his mother while they prepare dinner together.*

Assigning a Homework Task (Optional)

Goal discussion and/or exception questions can yield homework tasks for the family. In this case, the clinician reviews her perceptions of the family's problem. She can share these perceptions with the family or keep them to herself. This choice depends on whether she thinks that the family will benefit from an insight orientation. In this case she does, so she says that Ricky, like all children, needs attention from his parents. The dinner routine didn't seem to give him the attention he needed, but his "rude" behavior did gain their attention. Being sent to his room does temporarily stop the conflict but it doesn't get at the root of the problem: his need for attention. Finally, the father's and mother's parenting backgrounds are different and the father's "traditional" style is not working. Another approach is needed.

Clinician (referring to what was revealed by the exception questions): *Do you think you can do these things at home again—the sports talk and the pre-dinner talk?*

The family agrees.

Clinician: *Between now and our next meeting, I'd like you to practice each of those behaviors several times: Dad talking sports at the table, and Ricky helping Mom with dinner and sharing his school day with her or at the table.*

The clinician and the family review the specific behaviors in these interactions.

Clinician (preparing the family for a scaling question and measuring their feelings of hope): *I'd like to ask you all a different kind of question. On a scale of 1 to 10 with 1 being how hopeless you felt a few weeks ago when you called for the appointment and 10 being how you'd feel if you were to achieve your goal, where are you right now? Ricky, why don't you go first?*

Scaling Questions

The clinician asks each member a scaling question using the 1–10 scale.

Ricky: *I'd say about 5.*

Mother: *I'm at 7.*

Father: *Sounds like we're all doing better. I am at 6.*

Clinician (complimenting them and eliciting specific behaviors that helped them): *That's very impressive. What's helped you all get there?*

Ricky (smiling and "brightening" up): *Dad and I will talk about football.*

Father (demonstrating his insight and understanding): *I realize that Ricky wants attention just like I did when I was a kid. That helped.*

Mother: *I enjoy my time alone with Ricky.*

Scaling questions can yield homework tasks to help the family develop new patterns of interactions or revive past successful interactions.

Clinician (assigning homework tasks: using a scaling question to help each member develop a new behavior): *I am impressed by what you all have done. Let me ask another question. What would each of you have to do to move ahead on the scale by one number? For example, Ricky, what can you do to go from a 5 to a 6?*

Ricky: *I could quiz dad on some sports trivia.*

Mother: *I liked Ricky helping me at dinner.*

Clinician (helping the family appreciate the interactive context of achieving a new behavior): *Ricky, how could your mom help you go from a 5 to a 6?*

Ricky: *Letting me help her with dinner.*

Clinician (to father): *Is there some way you could help Ricky move to a 6? Tell Ricky.*

Father: *I could bring the sports page to the table as a reminder for us to talk about sports together.*

If the family can't readily think of other behaviors, the clinician can suggest some that fit the family's style and coping abilities.

Concluding the Meeting

The clinician summarizes the meeting, emphasizing the family's effort and achievements.

Clinician: *I'd like to take a minute and summarize all you've done—it's quite impressive. You were concerned about Ricky's rude behavior at the dinner table. You realized that several factors contributed to the problem. It wasn't just Ricky. You defined a family goal and developed some good solutions.*

The family was insightful, and the clinician did help the family members understand how their upbringings and ineffective responses influenced their dinnertime practices and affected their family relationships. She pointed out that Ricky did want attention and interactions through dinnertime conversation but that the "quiet" dinners thwarted this need and caused conflict. Sending him to his room isolated him and only intensified his need for attention.

The clinician helped the family remember its strengths by recalling past behaviors that had been successful. She used good discussion, exception questions, and scaling questions to help the family develop solutions.

The clinician used the family's insight to point out the interactive nature of the solution.

Clinician: *If Ricky can talk at the table, even for a short time, share his day, and get your attention and approval, then he's capable and willing to quiet down when asked. Ricky can change his behavior, but changing your behavior must also happen.*

Inviting the Family to Ask Questions or Share Thoughts

Clinician: *What questions or final thoughts would you like to share with me or with the family?*

Mother: *It felt good to sit here and talk instead of arguing, but I hope we don't forget what we did here.*

Clinician (using the homework tasks derived from the exception and scaling questions): *It is easy to forget. That's why I suggested you choose and practice a behavior at home; they're like reminders.*

Father: *I think we can do it.*

Clinician (reminding them of the family relationship aspect of changing their behavior): *But don't forget that you are not working alone. Everyone is working together and helping each other.*

Scheduling a Follow-up Visit

The clinician makes a follow-up appointment for 2 weeks.

Complimenting and Thanking the Family

Clinician: *Once again, congratulations on all you've done. Each of you contributed a lot. Thank you for coming in. I will see you soon.*

Post-Interview Phase

The clinician reviews the meeting. She feels satisfied with this first meeting because she had helped the family in the following ways:

- At the outset, she clearly stated that the meeting was family-oriented, not child-oriented.
- The clinician encouraged the family to discover and develop their own solutions.
  - Goal questions helped the family define and negotiate its own goals.
  - Exception questions helped the members rediscover past successes and reframe Ricky's behavior.
  - Scaling questions helped members measure their hope and competence and define new behaviors.

- She used family systems techniques.
  - The parenting history helped the parents understand how their past experiences influenced their present parenting practices.
  - She used insight-oriented questions and statements to help the family understand how repeating patterns of behavior maintained the problem and affected the family relationships.
  - The clinician helped the family develop specific behaviors to change the repeated patterns of interactions.
  - The clinician identified the father as the leader of the family and established an alliance with him.
  - The clinician reframed Ricky's behavior and helped the father change his perception of Ricky as a *"rude child"* to one of Ricky wanting to be a *"considerate child."*
- The clinician offered advice/teaching/reassurance.
  - She assigned homework tasks so the family could practice the new behaviors at home.
  - She explained Ricky's need for attention. The parents needed to help Ricky develop positive, not negative, behaviors to get their attention. They needed to change their behaviors too.
  - She set a follow-up date.

Chapter 26

The ABC Model

---

*T*he ABC interview (antecedent, behavior, consequence) highlights the "interactional context" of a parent–child behavioral problem. Invariably, child noncompliance, the most common parent complaint, is characterized by circular dynamics: the parent makes a request, the child responds/does not respond, the parent responds, the child responds, and so on. This pattern, which the ABC interview illustrates, can be repeated many times in a single incident (eg, *"I've told him six times to go to bed."*). These repetitive interactions rapidly become increasingly intense, maintain patterns of behavior, and leave both the child and parent feeling "stuck" (*"Nothing works."*) and frustrated (*"I've had it!"*).

"A" IS FOR THE *ANTECEDENT*

The antecedent is the "trigger" or situation that initiates child noncompliance. The trigger is part of the parent's communication and behavior—proximity to the child, parent's mood, actions, body language, word choice, eye contact, and/or facial expression. For example, the parent, with her hands on her hips, bends over the child while the child is reading a book and says impatiently, *"Come in the kitchen right now and do the dishes."*

"B" IS FOR *BEHAVIOR*

Behavior is the child's response to the trigger, which is the parent's request or command. It can be expressed by mood, actions, body language, word choice, eye contact, and/or facial expression. This is the identified "behavior problem." For example, the child could pause and initially pretend not to hear. Then he rolls his eyes, turns away from the mother, and answers in a sarcastic manner, *"Who do you think I am? Your servant? I don't want to."*

"C" IS FOR *CONSEQUENCE*

The consequence is the parent's reaction in response to the child's conduct. For example, the mother's demeanor is angry: her face reddens, her eyes narrow, her mouth tightens, and her lips purse. She reaches down; pulls the child up by his shirt; gets in his face; and responds in a shrill, strident voice, saying, *"How dare you talk to me like that. I work so hard and you treat me like a servant."* The parent's reaction affects the child, who responds to the mother more defiantly. She responds again with even more anger and attempts to drag him into the kitchen. This downward spiral can go on and on. It is hoped that the parents realize the futility of their circular, nonproductive interactions. The clinician can also ask *"What do you think would help?"* or *"Have there been other times when you did something else instead and things were better?"*

Once the clinician has an initial understanding of the problematic interactions, he or she can make suggestions and/or can help the family develop its own solutions. Figure 26.1 illustrates the ABC interview.

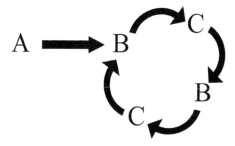

ABC Interview For Interactive Behaviors

A: Antecedent Event–Parent's Request or Command: Communication Style and Affect

B: Behavior–Child's Response to Parent: Behavior and Affect

C: Consequence–Parent's Response to Child: Behavior and Affect

BC: The Circular Dynamics Are Repeated and Form Parent-Child Interactive Patterns

Figure 26.1. ABC model.

INDICATIONS FOR USING THE ABC INTERVIEW

The ABC interview is useful as an initial interview for child noncompliance. Its use does not preclude exploration of the family context. Elements of the ABC interview can easily be combined with the solution-based interview or any other model.

The ABC interview follows the same sequence of steps as the other models outlined in this chapter. Initially, however, it focuses on the ABC interactions. More information (eg, a family history or recent family stresses) is gathered, as necessary, in subsequent interviews. An approximate timeframe of an ABC interview is listed in Box 26.1.

Box 26.1. The ABC–Antecedent, Behavior, Consequence–Interview: Steps and Questions

1. **Engaging the family** (time: 3–5 minutes)[a]
   Greet the family.
   Explain the purpose of the meeting.
2. **Understanding the family** (time: 10–15 minutes)[a]
   Define the problem.
   Use the ABC model.
   Understand the hierarchy.
   Identify family behaviors that maintain the problem.
3. **Working with the family** (time: 10–15 minutes)[a]
   Help the family cooperate in developing their own solutions.
   Offer advice when something unexpected happens.
4. **Concluding the meeting** (time: 3–5 minutes)[a]
   Summarize the meeting and answer questions.
   Ask the family for feedback.
   Schedule a follow-up visit.
   Compliment the family.

---

[a]These times are approximations based on the number of questions and complexity of the case.

Chapter 27

An Example of the ABC Model

―――――――――――■―――――――――――

CASE STUDY 27.1: THE FAMILY THAT IS "HAVING PROBLEMS" WITH THEIR 8-YEAR-OLD DAUGHTER

Mrs Greenwood calls to make an appointment because *"We're having problems with Pam."* The mother sounds very tense and says she wants *"a few minutes"* on the phone *"to explain the situation."* She makes so many references to *"we"* (the entire family) that the clinician suggests a family meeting. Mrs Greenwood says that she will ask her husband. She calls back to agree to a meeting.

Engaging the Family

Greeting the Family

The clinician reviews Pam's chart before the meeting. He has known her since she was a baby. The mother called her daughter *"strong-willed"* when she was a toddler. Otherwise, the chart contains nothing remarkable. The clinician knows little about the parents except that they seemed to be good and caring parents. The father owns a hardware store, and the mother is a hospital laboratory technician. After a cordial greeting and brief social conversation, the clinician explains the purpose of the meeting.

Explaining the Purpose of the Meeting

Clinician: *Mr and Mrs Greenwood, have you explained to Pam why we are meeting?*

Father: *Not really.*

Clinician: *Pam, do you know why we are meeting?*

Pam: *My problem.*

Clinician: *What does "my problem" mean?*

Pam: *That's what Mommy said.*

Mother: *It seems that we are bumping heads all the time and can't seem to get along and it's very stressful.*

Clinician: *Pam, do you think that is an issue?*

Pam: *I suppose it is because nobody seems happy now.*

Clinician (removing the blame focus from Pam and emphasizing the family context): *Pam, no one is blaming you. We're meeting to talk about a family concern and, most of all, to help you and Mom and Dad get along better. Everyone is going to work together.*

Pam does not look up or respond. The clinician allows a silence of about 10 seconds and then speaks.

Clinician: *How does that sound to you?*

Pam: *All right, I guess.*

The clinician isn't sure if Pam understands or agrees with this shift to a family orientation. She tries again.

Clinician (deciding to avoid the word "problem"): *Sometimes families are not happy and need help. We are here to make your family happy...you, Mom, Dad, and I need the whole family to talk and work together to make that happen. Would you like to try?*

Pam: *I think so.*

Clinician (to parents): *How about you?*

The parents nod vigorously.

Clinician (to Pam): *Can you talk with us and help us?*

Pam: *I'll try.*

Clinician: *Good for you.*

The clinician has explained the purpose carefully, and Pam is willing to try. When the clinician compliments Pam, he looks at the parents, hoping they will respond. They get the hint and compliment Pam too. The clinician did this because he wanted to bring out a positive quality in Pam and to lessen the "problem" focus of the meeting.

UNDERSTANDING THE FAMILY AND ITS CONCERN

Defining the Problem

Clinician: *I know we spoke on the phone, Mrs Greenwood, but let's review your concern again to be sure that it's clear to everyone and that you all agree.*

To reduce any feelings of blame, the clinician avoids the "problem."

Mother: *Every day I call her for breakfast and she dawdles until the morning is ruined.*

Clinician (seeking clarification and also confronting): *Ruined?*

Father: *We are upset. We eat in 2 minutes. We rush to work and school. It's a bad way to start the day.*

Clinician (getting Pam's input so the interview is not dominated by the parents' problem talk): *Pam, what do you want to say?*

Pam: *They yell at me. I don't like that.*

Clinician: *It sounds like arriving late for breakfast and then having everyone get "upset" are the issues. Is that right?*

Father: *That's right.*

Mother: *If Pam could just get ready....*

Clinician (intentionally preventing the mother from resuming problem talk): *Let's find out what the family is doing in the morning.*

USING THE ABC MODEL

Antecedent

The next step for the clinician is to obtain a very clear, specific description of the antecedent, or "A," aspect of the ABC model.

Clinician (to parents): *I'd like you to think of the specific instance in which this situation occurs. Give us an example of how you ask Pam to come, including your words, tone of voice, and location when you are asking Pam.*

Mother: *"Pam, come down for breakfast." My tone of voice is pleasant. Of course, she can't see me because I am in the kitchen and she's upstairs in her bedroom, so I do have to raise my voice.*

Clinician (determining the father's involvement): *Mr Greenwood, where are you and what are you doing at this time?*

Father: *I'm usually in our bedroom watching the morning news. I just have a bagel and coffee for breakfast so I get downstairs a few minutes later. I do step into the hallway to tell Pam, "You heard what your mother said." That's my routine.*

Clinician: *Pam, what are you doing?*

Pam: *I'm watching TV in my room.*

Clinician: *How are you all feeling when this part happens?*

They report that they are all feeling *"okay."*

Behavior

Next the clinician explores the parents' complaint, which is usually the child's problematic behavior (the "B" aspect of the ABC model). He wants to know the child's response to the parents' request or command, which is the behavior that the parents want to change. The clinician asks Pam and her parents to describe her behavior briefly (actions, words, and emotions) and to establish a baseline measure (eg, frequency [number of incidents daily or weekly] and/or duration [how long a single incident lasts]). The measure will allow them to negotiate a reasonable goal (eg, 20% improvement in several weeks, 1 day a week when things are better).

Clinician: *Pam, when Mom calls you, what do you do?*

Pam: *I don't hear Mom.*

Clinician: *Do you hear Dad?*

Pam: *Sometimes.*

Clinician: *What do you do?*

Pam: *I keep watching TV.*

Clinician (to parents): *Is that the concern?*

Mother: *That's it. She doesn't answer me and doesn't come to breakfast.*

Father: *I know she hears me, but she stays in her room.*

Clinician: *How often does this happen, and how long does one incident last?*

The parents state that it happens *"every school day"* and lasts about 5 minutes *"until we blow up."*

Consequence

The clinician should next explore the consequence (the "C" in the ABC model) or the parental response to the child's initial behavior (B). The clinician would ask the parent(s) to describe his or her (their) actions, words, and emotions. For example, the parent's response might include repeating the requests, threatening (*"I'll tell your father."*), giving up (*"Oh well, it doesn't really matter."*), postponing (*"We'll talk about this tomorrow."*), doing the task alone (*"It's easier to do it myself."*), or scolding the child (*"You are being so rude."*).

Clinician (to mother): *Tell us how you respond when Pam stays in her room.*

Mother: *I raise my voice and repeat the command several times in short succession. I yell at my husband to bring her down.*

Clinician (to parents): *How does each of you feel when Pam stays in her room?*

Mother: *I am angry with both of them because I'm trying to fix breakfast and get ready for work and Pam doesn't come when I call her. I yell at him to bring her to breakfast.*

Father: *I raise my voice too and tell Pam to get downstairs. I'm losing patience with her, but I'm trying to see the end of the news report. I also don't like my wife yelling at me. So I'm upset at both of them.*

The clinician realizes how each member's behaviors contribute to the problem. The mother is now trying both to get Pam to breakfast and to enlist her husband's support, and both parents are getting upset at Pam and at each other.

The clinician explores the next cycle of the child–parent interaction, another cycle of B and C.

Clinician: *Pam, do you hear Mom and Dad now? What do you do?*

Pam: *I hear Mom and Dad, and I start to get ready.*

Clinician (seeking clarification): *Ready?*

Pam: *I still watch TV because I know Mom or Dad will come and get me.*

Clinician: *How are you feeling at this time?*

Pam: *Okay.*

Clinician (to parents): *What happens next?*

Mother: *I am exasperated by now. I stomp upstairs to Pam's room, turn off the TV, and tell her "Now!" I know I have a mean expression on my face.*

Pam: *Mom's face is red.*

Father: *When I hear her coming up the stairs, I turn off my TV and go to Pam's room. I try to help out by calming my wife, but she's fussing at me and at Pam. I'm upset with Pam too, but also with my wife for losing her temper again.*

Clinician: *Pam, now how do you feel?*

Pam: *Sometimes I feel scared.*

At this point, Pam begins to cry. Her mother takes her on her lap and comforts her.

Father: *It gets pretty intense some days, especially if we are running late for the school bus and work. But sometimes Pam gets kind of mad, yells back at her mother or me, and says she doesn't want breakfast. Then one of us brings her downstairs. Once at the table, she usually eats something although she's pouting.*

Clinician: *Do you spank her or grab her?*

Mother: *Never. Neither one of us. But sometimes, I do feel like giving her a "pop" on her rear end.*

Clinician: *Thank you for telling this story. It helped me understand the family behavior.*

UNDERSTANDING THE HIERARCHY

The clinician still is not sure who was in charge of getting Pam downstairs.

Clinician: *Who's in charge of the morning routine?*

Mother: *I am, but I can't do it all.*

Father: *Sometimes I feel like Pam is in control. She makes it happen.*

Clinician (attempting to remove the blame from Pam and to change the father's perception): *It seems like there is a lot going on. Everyone is affected. It's not just Pam.*

The clinician wonders who is in charge. The mother is taking on too much. She is making breakfast, packing Pam's lunch, and trying to get Pam and her father down for breakfast. Maybe the father could be in charge of Pam. The clinician decides to raise that issue later in the interview (see Working With the Family below).

IDENTIFYING FAMILY PATTERNS THAT MAINTAIN THE PROBLEM

Now that the family has described the problematic interactions, the clinician reviews the series of behaviors, hoping the family members might better understand how each of their behaviors maintain the problem. However, the clinician must realize that this insight-oriented task will not work with all families.

Clinician: *Can you see how the family's interactions tend to prolong the problem? Everyone is stuck in the same pattern, and it's very hard to break out and try something new.*

Mother: *It seems like we're all caught up in this together. I used to think she was just being stubborn, but it's not that simple.*

Father: *We just go round and round and get nowhere.*

The family's responses are insightful and indicate that the members are ready to make changes in their morning routine.

Clinician (demystifying the situation in a supportive manner): *Again, let me emphasize that no one is to blame. It's just that your responses, which are to work harder, louder, and longer, just aren't working. You need to find another way. All three of you need to be in charge of making a change. How does that sound to you?*

Family (father, mother, and Pam): *We agree.*

WORKING WITH THE FAMILY

The clinician helps the family cooperate to develop its own solutions.

Clinician (helping the family change the situation and its behavior in the Antecedent with a modified goal question): *How can you work together to improve things? For example, how could the first situation, when Mom first calls Pam to the table, be improved?*

Mother: *It's probably true that she can't hear me. Maybe I should go to her room.*

Father: *That's fine. I could help out by turning off my TV and getting Pam when I hear you call.*

Mother: *Maybe Pam's door could stay open, so she would hear me.*

Clinician (helping the family change its interactions in the next phase): *Pam, is there anything you could do to get down to breakfast on time?*

Pam: *I don't know.*

Clinician: *Pam, could you think of something you could do?*

Pam: *I'll try hard to come to breakfast when called.*

Father: *I could bring Pam downstairs with me.*

The father has "volunteered" to help be in charge of Pam. This change of role removes the mother from her repetitive patterns with Pam and lessens the burden on her. The father's offer signals a very important and positive change that clearly demonstrates his support for his wife. This change alone, if carried out successfully, will improve the family functioning.

THE FAMILY'S OWN IDEAS WORK BEST

When families come up with their own ideas and solutions, they are more likely to work than if the clinician suggests them.

Clinician: *Are you saying you will be in charge of Pam? That would let your wife be in charge of making breakfast and lunch only. Tell her.*

Father (looking at his wife): *I'm willing to try.*

Clinician (acknowledging the mother as leader and gauging whether she will agree): *Can you go along with that? Tell him.*

Mother (holding on to her power and reluctant to try this): *I'm not sure if you can come through.*

Clinician (gently persuading the mother to trust the father): *Do you think you could let go a bit and allow your husband and Pam to try it together? Tell them what you think.*

Mother (looking at the family): *If it would make things easier, let's try it.*

Father (stepping up to his new role and asking Pam to consider how she might change her behavior): *Pam, how can you help out?*

Pam: *By coming downstairs with you when Mom calls.*

Mother (assuming her proper role in the hierarchy): *I also want no TV in the mornings.*

Sometimes families have unrealistic expectations or want to change things too fast. In this case, the mother is asking for too much change at once.

Clinician (helping the family set a realistic goal): *How much improvement would you like to see in the next 2 weeks?*

Mother (looking at her husband and Pam): *We all need to improve our behavior, but let's be realistic. If Pam and her dad came down together twice a week, that would be a good start. If I have to call out again, which I probably will at times, I will walk upstairs and tell him. I will try to remember not to yell.*

Clinician (to Pam and the father): *Does that sound like a workable plan?*

OFFERING ADVICE/SUPPORT WHEN SOMETHING UNEXPECTED HAPPENS

Mother: *I have a last thought. I think we might remove the TV from Pam's room. It is such a distraction, and she watches silly cartoons.*

Father: *I don't agree.*

At this point, Pam breaks into tears, hops off her mother's lap, and sits in her own chair.

For a parent to suddenly "add on" another problem or request at the end of a visit is not unusual. The clinician should politely postpone this agenda and offer to address it in the next meeting. The goal is to get agreement on one behavior and not get distracted by another at this meeting.

Clinician (respecting this new concern, but wanting to preserve the family's sense of accomplishment, and knowing this was not the time to address another issue, like TV, says the following): *With all due respect, I'd like to suggest that you not try anything else at this time. You've done a lot of work here and have a lot to practice at home. The TV viewing is obviously an issue. I am not dismissing it, but I think we can address it at our next meeting.*

CONCLUDING THE MEETING

Summarizing the Meeting and Answering Questions

Clinician: *This has been a very productive meeting. Through your open and honest conversation, you have seen how everyone can help a family issue/ concern keep going and how everyone can help end it by changing roles and behaviors. You've come up with a realistic goal and a good plan.*

Mother: *I'm not convinced that it's going to work. Can we call you if we have problems?*

Clinician: *Certainly. Now, what questions or comments would you like to share with one another?*

Pam: *Does that mean I can still have my TV?*

Mother (being more patient and offering alternatives): *For the time being. We'll discuss that at our next meeting. Maybe you could earn TV time.*

Asking the Family for Feedback

Clinician: *I'd like to ask you how the meeting went for you. Did it help you address your concerns?*

The family feels it has been a *"good start."*

Clinician: *How do you feel now compared to when you came in?*

Father: *A little bit better.*

Pam: *What do you mean?*

Clinician: *Do you feel better now than before?*

Pam: *I think so.*

Mother: *I'm not sure. I'll tell you at the next meeting.*

Clinician (to the father): *Mr Greenwood, let's hear from you.*

Father: *This is a good start. Finally, we're moving forward.*

Scheduling a Follow-up Visit

The clinician schedules a follow-up appointment in 2 weeks.

Complimenting the Family

Clinician: *I want to tell you how well you worked together. It's apparent you really want to change the morning routine. Each of you came up with a behavior that working together on should help make a change. I hope you can practice at home what you discussed here. Thank you for coming in.*

THE POST-INTERVIEW PHASE

The clinician reviews the meeting. He had done several different things.
- He explained the purpose of a family meeting.
- He used the ABC model to show families the circular nature of a "behavioral problem."
- He helped the family break their negative pattern of behavior and to develop its own solutions. Most importantly, the father "volunteered" to take on a new role/behavior and to support his wife. This is a key change.
- The clinician used several family systems techniques.
  — He illustrated the interactive context/relationship aspects of the problem.
  — He identified family interactions that maintain the problem.
  — He explored the hierarchy and identified the mother as the leader.
  — He helped the family discuss its own ways to change its behaviors/interactive patterns.
- The clinician offered advice/support.
  — He gently urged the mother to relinquish some power, to drop one responsibility, and to agree with her husband's desire to assume some power/leadership. This agreement is a major change.
  — He raised the issue of setting realistic expectations, and the mother responded with a realistic goal.
  — He postponed the discussion of removing the TV from Pam's room because it would probably have "undone" all the good work the family had accomplished. He did this respectfully and did acknowledge its importance to the family by promising to discuss it later.

— He complimented the family and reminded it of its homework assignments.
— He dictated a summary letter to the family and used a copy as his chart note.

SECTION E SUMMARY

This section described 5 conceptual models of family interviewing: Satir's communication model, Minuchin's structural family model, Haley's problem-solving model, the brief solution-oriented model, and the ABC model. Examples of each model are listed below. Each model has been illustrated with a case study. Pediatric care professionals (PCPs) often select and combine various aspects of different models. They also may individualize the interviewing techniques to best fit their own particular styles; their time constraints; their office policies; and the family's issues, style, and values. Case studies were used to illustrate these models.

Examples of Models

- **Satir**
  — There are various determinants of communication and behavioral interactions (eg, family structure and function, roles, rules, and biological determinants).
  — Communication patterns may be functional or dysfunctional: functional promotes clarification and self-validation, dysfunctional is invalidating and conflicting.
  — Both sender and receiver are responsible for clear communication.
  — Parents need to understand levels of child language development.
  — Many examples of common communication problems and solutions are described.
- **Minuchin**
  — Family systems: a system or organization that functions through repeated interactive behaviors, which determine how and when members interact and relate.
  — Family subsystems: various subsystems exist within each family (eg, the parent subsystem, spousal/partner subsystem, and sibling subsystem). Subsystems are separated and distinguished by boundaries.
  — Boundaries: a collection of rules (spoken and unspoken) that dictate who participates and their manner of participating in a particular subsystem. For example, the parental subsystem defines participants and their power, roles, and behavior. Boundaries may be diffuse, rigid, or clear/appropriate.
  — Hierarchy: the power structure that defines leadership and authority and how authority is asserted. The clinician must always identify the leader of a hierarchy.

- **Haley**
  - Problem-solving: based on defining roles, assigning roles, constructing an intervention within the family's coping abilities and social situation.
  - The PCP must determine when to give advice and suggestions. The family must be rational and have control, but sometimes "good advice" does not work if the family is not ready for it.
  - Problem-solving assumes that family members interact in predictable, repetitive patterns based on the family's organizational pattern.
  - These directives must be specific, realistic, meaningful, and achievable.
- **Solution-Oriented Model**
  - This model focuses more on construction of solutions than on problem talk.
  - Solution talk has 3 major components: goal definition and discussion, exception questions, and scaling questions.
  - The focus is to help families work together to achieve realistic goals, define each member's role, and emphasize the interactive context of solution building.
- **ABC Model**
  - This model demonstrates the circular and reciprocal nature of relationships and behavioral concerns.
    - Antecedent event
    - Behavior
    - Consequence
  - Antecedent is the parent behavior ("trigger"), such as a suggestion or command that precipitates a response in the child.
  - Behavior is the child's response or nonresponse to the parental request or command.
  - Consequence is the parent's response to the child's initial response.
  - Behavior and consequence continue to affect each other in a cyclical, repetitive manner.

Skills Checklist

- Review the names and central concepts of each of the 5 models of family interviewing.
- Review the various components of each of the 5 models of family interviewing.
- Discuss how a PCP can pick and choose various components of the models and integrate them into his or her interview.
- Discuss the factors that might determine how a PCP selects and uses these components to promote a "fit" between the style of the PCP and that of the family.
- Discuss your own cases and how you might apply components of these models.

SUGGESTED READING

Allmond BW, Tanner JL. *The Family Is the Patient*. Baltimore, MD: Lippincott, Williams & Wilkins; 1999

Baker B, Brightman A, Heifetz L, et al. *Behavior Problems*. Champaign, IL: Research Press; 1976

Barker P. *Basic Family Therapy*. 3rd ed. New York, NY: Oxford University Press; 1992

Berg IK. *Family-Based Services*. New York, NY: Norton; 1994

Coleman WL. Family-focused pediatrics: solution-oriented techniques for behavioral problems. *Contemp Pediatr*. 1997;14:121–134

DeShazer S. *Keys to Solution in Brief Therapy*. New York, NY: WW Norton; 1985

Doherty WJ, Baird MA. *Family Therapy and Family Medicine*. New York, NY: Guilford Press; 1983

Faber A, Maylish E. *How to Talk so Kids Will Listen and Listen so Kids Will Talk*. New York, NY: Avon Books; 1980

Haley J. *Problem Solving Therapy*. San Francisco, CA: Jossey-Bass; 1987

King M, Novik L, Citrenbaum C. *Irresistible Communication: Creative Skills for the Health Professional*. Philadelphia, PA: WB Saunders; 1983

Klar H, Coleman WL. Brief solution-focused strategies for behavioral pediatrics. *Pediatr Clin North Am*. 1995;42(1):131–141

McKay M, Davis M, Fanning P. *How to Communicate*. New York, NY: MJF Books; 1983

Minuchin S, Fishman H. *Family Therapy Techniques*. Cambridge, MA: Harvard University Press; 1981

Nichols MP, Schwartz RC. *Family Therapy: Concepts and Methods*. 2nd ed. New York, NY: Allyn and Bacon; 1991

Satir V. *Conjoint Family Therapy*. Palo Alto, CA: Science and Behavior Books; 1972

Satir V. *The New People Making*. Mountain View, CA: Science and Behavior Books; 1983

Selekman MD. *Solution-Focused Therapy With Children*. New York, NY: Guilford Press; 1997

Walsh F. *Strengthening Family Resilience*. New York, NY: Guilford Press; 1998

Walter JL, Peller JE. *Becoming Solution-Focused in Brief Therapy*. New York, NY: Brunner/Mazel; 1992

Whiteside-Mansell L, Bradely RH, McKelvey L, Fussell JJ. Parenting: linking impacts of interpartner conflict to preschool children's social behavior. *J Pediatr Nurs*. 2009;24(5):389–400

Techniques for Assessing and Enhancing Family Functioning

*T*here are many ways to assess and enhance family functioning. This section describes 3 categories
1. Observing the family activities in the meeting
2. Gathering more information by more interviewing
3. Offering suggestions to the family

Chapter 28

Observing Family Activities in the Meeting

Observing family activities in the meeting is to assign tasks and watch how the family carries them out. Examples of activities are listed in Box 28.1 and described below.

> ### Box 28.1. Five Techniques for Observing Families in Assigned Tasks
> 1. Family draws a picture together
> 2. Child draws a picture
> 3. Role-playing
> 4. Hand puppets
> 5. Magic wand

FAMILY DRAWS A PICTURE TOGETHER

The family drawing lets the clinician observe the nonverbal family interaction. The game-like feeling of this activity helps young children and/or hesitant, less verbal family members relax and get involved. In the 5 to 10 minutes allotted for this brief activity, the clinician observes both the content (what each member draws) and the process (how they share space, communicate, cooperate, and follow the directions) of the drawing.

For the activity, the family sits at a table and is given a large sheet of paper. Each member chooses a single crayon of a different color.

The clinician gives the family directions in the following way:

Clinician: *I would like each of you to draw something. You may draw whatever you want. Please don't talk to anyone, including me, during this exercise. You have 5 minutes.*

Observing Family Interactions

The clinician observes the family interactions during the process. When time is up, the clinician asks each member to describe his or her drawing (content). The clinician encourages members to comment on the process: how he or she interacted, how others interacted, and the feelings he or she experienced. The clinician may ask the following questions:

- *"How did you decide to draw what you drew?"*
- *"How did others draw theirs?"*
- *"Were you working together or alone?"*
- *"Would you like to have done it differently?"*
- *"What were you feeling during this task (game)?"*

From the activity and responses, the clinician gains initial, general impressions about the family interactions. The clinician notes what others drew and asks similar questions to the other family members. One must emphasize and remember that these conclusions are only preliminary and thus they may be confirmed or altered as the clinician learns more about the family. Below are some observations and their possible interpretations (in parentheses).

- Did the family members draw thick lines to enclose their space (rigid boundaries) or give "intruders" (those who draw in their "space") a stern look ("forbids" others to enter)?
- Did they "hide" their drawing from others (keep secrets, want privacy, avoid criticism)?
- Did individual members extend their drawings (a ray of sunshine, a tree branch, a straight line) into others' space (reaches out, invites others to cooperate)?
- Did members make eye contact, smile, and want others to look at their drawing (open, friendly, shares, wants praise)?
- Did members look at others' drawings and smile and nod (approving, accepting)?
- Did they scowl and grimace when looking at the drawings of others (disapproving, rejecting)?
- Did they begin right away (initiative, confidence)?
- Did they wait and watch before beginning (hesitancy, dependency)?
- Did one member act as a leader and the others as followers (hierarchy)?
- Did any members seem to join together against another (coalition)?
- Did any members work together in a positive manner (alliance)?

CHILD DRAWS A PICTURE OF THE FAMILY

Having the child draw a picture of the family provides an opportunity for the child to describe his or her feelings and perceptions about himself or herself, family members, and family problems. To start this activity, the clinician gives the child a piece of paper (on a clipboard or table) and a single crayon, pencil, or felt-tip pen. The clinician instructs the child by saying, *"Draw a picture of you and your family doing something."* While the child draws the picture, the clinician speaks with the parents, observes how the child carries out the task (the process), and assesses if the child

- Works independently
- Pesters the parent
- Needs reassurance
- Experiences any particular feeling(s)

The clinician also observes how the parents respond to the child during this process. Did they allow the child to work independently or did they help and advise the child?

The clinician then asks the child about the content.

- *"What did you draw?"*
- *"Can you tell us about your drawing?"*
- *"Who are the people?"*
- *"What are they doing?"*
- *"How are they feeling"*

The clinician encourages the following responses from the parents:

- Sharing their reactions to the child's drawing
- Asking questions about the child's drawing
- Complimenting the child on his or her picture
- Being nonjudgmental and empathetic toward the child

ROLE-PLAYING

Role-playing allows the parent and child to reenact a problematic interaction, to practice a desired interaction, and to express related emotions. For some families, role-playing "breaks the ice" and helps them shift to a family focus. For example, a mother might present with the chief complaint that *"the child doesn't mind me."* After a few minutes of problem description and goal negotiation, the clinician asks the mother and daughter to role-play a difficult interaction that occurs regularly.

- **The problem**

  Clinician: *I need you to help me understand the issue better. I'd like to have each of you pretend you are home. I'd like you* (mother) *to enter Susan's* (daughter) *room and ask her to pick up her clothes. And then Susan, I want you to act like you do when Mom asks you to clean up your room. I'd like you both to act and talk and look and sound just like you do at home. I'll help you.*

- **The thoughts and feelings associated with the problem.** After a few minutes of role-playing the problematic situation, the clinician asks the mother and daughter to discuss their actions, the others' actions, and their feelings.

Clinician: *What were you doing or trying to do? What was Mom doing? How did each of you feel? How do you think the other person was feeling?*

- **The desired interaction.** In this use of the technique, the clinician asks the mother and daughter to describe their goal or what they'd like to happen.

  Clinician: *Now let's go through this again but now both of you act and talk in a way to make your goal happen.*

- **The feelings associated with the new desired interaction.** After a few minutes of role-playing the desired behavior, the clinician asks the mother and daughter to discuss their feelings as they role-played their goal behavior.

  Clinician: *How did each of you feel now? How do you think the other was feeling?*

- **To promote the interactive aspect**

  Clinician: *How could Mom help you do better? How could you help Mom to act in a happier way with you?*

HAND PUPPETS

Like role-playing, hand puppets can be used to re-create a problematic inter-action, to rehearse a desired interaction, and to communicate associated feel-ings. Members can either play themselves or assume the identity of the hand puppet (eg, a bear, a clown, or an identity of their own choice). Acting as a "character" instead of as oneself often makes expressing oneself easier (for children especially) because the individual can pretend he or she is someone else in this "make believe" game. The hand puppet game should be conducted like the role-playing exercise.

MAGIC WAND

The magic wand provides an easy, effective way to help children express their feelings, thoughts, or wishes. This activity works well with children because they think imaginatively and express themselves more easily by playing and making wishes. This activity helps the clinician and the parents understand their feelings, therefore promoting a family discussion. The magic wand, which can be purchased in most toy stores, is a clear plastic tube filled with clear oil and little bits of sparkle, stars, moons, or other figures. The clinician does not even need to use a real wand; a pen or pencil can be substituted and the clinician can instruct the child to *"pretend this is a magic wand."*

The clinician would conduct this activity in the following ways:

- The clinician hands the magic wands to the child and parent(s) and says (asking the child to go first), *"Now wave the magic wand and make a wish."*
- The clinician asks the child to make a general wish or a wish that is more specific to the child's or family's needs. The clinician could say, *"Make a wish about what you would like to see happen at home,"* or *"Make a wish about what would make you happy."*
- The clinician encourages the child to hold the wand and to express their feelings. The clinician could ask, *"When you made that wish what were you feeling?"*
- The clinician now repeats the steps with the parent.
- The clinician uses the child's wish to initiate a family discussion. The clinician starts the discussion with a statement, like *"Ms Miller, what do you think about Sandra's wish?"* or *"How did you feel when you heard Sandra's wish?"* The clinician then asks Sandra, *"What do you think about Mom's wish?"*
- The clinician invites other members to wave the wand and make a wish. Other members often participate to be supportive of the child, but it also allows them to share their wishes and feelings with the rest of the family in a nonthreatening way.

Chapter 29

Gathering More Information by Further Interviewing

*H*aving too much information can easily overwhelm the clinician. However, often assessing all components of family functioning is not necessary. Gathering it all in one meeting is certainly not feasible.

To gather more information about family functioning, the clinician should decide what would be most helpful. Five other sources of information are described in this chapter. They were not included in the descriptions of the family interview. Family history, for example, provides essential information, whereas information from the family life cycle may be lower priority. See Box 29.1.

Box 29.1. Other Techniques to Assess Family Functioning

1. Family history
2. Stressors and support
3. Parenting history
4. Family life cycle
5. Brief family genogram

FAMILY HISTORY

The family history (eg, medical and psychosocial history) provides valuable information about family functioning.

The following principles guide the clinician in exploring family history:

- Explore after a good relationship with the family has been established.
- Remember that the exploration does not have to be completed in one visit.
- Introduce it in a respectful manner that emphasizes its importance. The clinician might say, *"I'd like to ask a few questions about your physical and mental health and the health of other family members. This will help me understand the family. I ask these questions with all families."*

Family history has many components, some of which families are used to (questions about medical problems—cancer, hypertension) and which are not perceived as threatening or intrusive. However, necessary inquiries about mental health and personal problems are more sensitive to the family and sometimes are perceived as intrusive or irrelevant. Therefore, the clinician should start with medical illnesses before psychosocial issues.

Medical Illness

The clinician can inquire about grandparents, aunts, uncles, and any other relative as well as immediate family. Questioning might begin as follows, *"Let's start with you, the parents. Do either of you have medical problems? Are you receiving care? How have these problems affected you and your family?"*

Psychosocial Problems

- **Behavior problems.** Specific questions to ask include, *"Does your child remind you of yourself or of another relative?" "How would you describe your behavior as a child or teenager?"* and *"Did you or any relatives have any problems?" "Did this person get help? Was it helpful?"*
- **Mental health problems.** The clinician can use the parent's concern (eg, child depression) as a way to inquire about family history. Queries can include, *"Have you or any relative ever been diagnosed with anxiety, depression, or any other mental health problem?" "Was treatment suggested?" "What kind of treatment was suggested?" "Medication?" "Counseling?" "Was it helpful?"* and *"How has this affected you and your family?"*
- **Alcohol or drug problems.** Examples of questions include, *"Have you or another family member ever had a problem with alcohol or drug use either now or in the past?" "Have you or another family member received help? Was it helpful?"* and *"How has this affected you and your family?"*

If parents state they are currently affected by any of these problems, the clinician should **always** ask if they are getting treatment and if it is helpful. If the treatment is not helpful or if parents who wish to receive treatment are not getting it, the clinician can offer assistance by suggesting a referral in the following way:

Clinician: *Would you be interested in getting help? Do you have a primary care provider who could help or who could make a referral? Would you like me to help with a referral?*

STRESSORS AND SUPPORTS

Stressors and supports are influences that negatively or positively affect family functioning. They can be internal (within the family) and/or external (outside the family). Although the clinician does not have to explore all possible stressors and supports, he or she should explore issues that are raised by the family or that the clinician thinks are relevant.

Below are several examples of how to inquire about stresses and supports. For example, if a parent spontaneously states, *"This problem has really affected my marriage,"* the clinician might ask, *"How has it affected your marriage?" "How would you describe your marriage?"* or *"Have you considered getting help?"*

External stressors can include lack of transportation to attend an appointment at the clinic or hospital or lack of access to health care. In these cases the clinician might refer the family to a hospital or to the county Department of Social Services. Some internal stressors might include the same problems the clinician finds with a family history; however, both the clinician and the family might feel that discussing "stressors" instead of "family history" is easier. The use of "stressors" is often perceived as less intrusive and less personal. Other stressors might include marital discord or domestic violence.

More families are serving in the military with an increased risk for mental health problems in fathers and mothers, which affect the entire family. Pediatric care professionals (PCPs) should inquire about mental health problems in all families, but especially families at risk, such as military families (depression, anxiety, acute stress reactions, and sleep disorders).

The clinician can help the family feel comfortable in answering these questions by making a statement such as, *"Every family experiences stress from time to time. I'd like to ask if you or a relative/partner has experienced any stresses or changes recently, especially around the time that the problems started."*

If the family seems hesitant or unsure in response to this question, the clinician can follow with a more specific question such as, *"For example, has anyone experienced any new stress recently, like changes at work or drinking problems at home?"* or *"Has anyone tried to find help for this issue?"*

The clinician should always search for supports and stressors. Supports would include a supportive social network, friends and family, religious organizations, community resources, medical resources, and adequate income (Box 29.2).

Box 29.2. Recording Stresses and Supports

Directions: Use "–" if a stressor and "+" if a strength. The absence of a support may be considered a stressor.

Extended family _____   Housing _____   Income _____

Friends _____   Schools _____   Employment/career _____

Neighborhood _____   Transportation _____   Social services _____

Cultural system _____   Recreational resources _____   Health care _____

Religion _____   (physical and mental)

Family goals and plans

Strengths and Supports	Stressors and Risk Factors
1.	1.
2.	2.
3.	3.
4.	4.

Comments:

PARENTING HISTORY

Asking parents about their upbringing and the ways that they were raised helps the clinician understand their parenting practices and beliefs. Parents' tendencies are to treat their children as they themselves were treated. A brief discussion between the parents and the clinician often gives both parties insight into how and why the parents act the way they do toward their children. With this understanding, changing parenting practices and parent–parent or parent–child interactions are 2 of the most common goals in family counseling. When parents reflect about their own upbringing, they often gain insight into their own parenting practices. Sometimes this understanding alone motivates them to change undesirable practices and habits.

The clinician should first explain the reason for asking the parents about their parenting history. An example of how to do so follows.

Clinician: *The way we were raised as children strongly influences how we raise our own children. I'd like to ask you a few questions about your parents and how they raised you.*

The questions are intended to elicit descriptions of the following components of parenting style:
- Expression and demonstration of positive and negative emotions
- Openness of communication
- Amount of parenting control

Questions regarding expression and demonstration of positive emotions (affection, pride, warmth, acceptance, approval, and love) and negative emotions (withholding affection, belittling, humiliating, criticizing, scolding, nagging, blaming) include
- *"Did your own parents readily express their love, pleasure, and approval? Their displeasure?"*
- *"How did they show these feelings?"*
- *"Did they give you praise and encouragement?"*
- *"How would you describe your relationship with your mother? Father? Siblings?"*

Questions regarding openness of communication (thoughts and feelings) between parents and children include
- *"How did your parents communicate with you?"*
- *"Did they encourage you to express your feelings and thoughts?"*
- *"Were some topics or feelings never discussed?"*
- *"How does that affect you and your communication with your children?"*
- *"Would you like to have more open communication with your children?"*
- *"How did your parents resolve their conflicts (settle their arguments) between themselves or with you?"*

In the area of amount of parental control, "control" can range from restrictive/controlling/highly supervised to lax/permissive/loosely supervised. Questions include
- *"How would you describe your parents' main parenting style?"*
- *"Were they strict? Permissive? In between?"*
- *"What were your parents' shortcomings and strengths?"*
- *"How do their behaviors and parenting styles affect you and your children?"*
- *"How did your parents reward you or acknowledge good effort and behavior?"*
- *"How did they punish you or show disapproval for undesirable behaviors?"*
- *"Were they fair?"*

- *"Did your mother and father have different parenting styles? How did they resolve their differences?"*
- *"Do you parent differently from your parents? Does your style work for your family now?"*

FAMILY LIFE CYCLE

All families grow through stages of development: the family life cycle. For most families, it is a series of normal transitions and transformations that follow a predictable pattern: marriage or a committed relationship, the birth of children, children and adolescents and then adult children, middle years, old age, and finally death. Specific developmental tasks are accomplished in each transition. Exploring the family's stage in the life cycle provides much information about the family.

Family life cycle changes, such as becoming a family with adolescents or with elderly grandparents, require adjustments that can be stressful. These changes are internal stressors or "growing pains of families." Although families respond to help and guidance with these changes, the stresses of these transitional phases are often temporary and thus are not necessarily indicative of serious dysfunction. The clinician should use the family life cycle to pinpoint the family's stage of development in order to help the parents understand and adapt to the challenges facing them. Many families cope well with these transitions unless additional changes are imposed on the family life cycle (eg, internal stressors, such as divorce or the formation of a stepfamily, or external stressors, such as the loss of a job or the move to a new city or state). Then the family's coping ability may be overwhelmed. The clinician can use the family life cycle to help the family members understand the expectations and challenges facing them at this particular point in their own family life cycle. The clinician should review the family's stage in the life cycle.

An example of appropriate questioning for the arrival of a baby appears below.

- *The arrival of a baby*
  - What developmental task/challenge most affects the family?
  - How are new parents adjusting to their new parent roles?
  - Are they learning to share the parenting responsibilities?
  - What else is happening in the lives of the parents, grandparents, and other children (if the family includes older children)?
    - **Parents**
      - ◆ Describe their physical and social–emotional health.
      - ◆ How are they doing with their marriage/partner relationship and jobs?
      - ◆ How is their relationship with their parents?
      - ◆ Do they have a support network?

- **Grandparents**
  - ◆ Describe their physical and social–emotional health.
  - ◆ If they have problems (eg, physical, emotional, or social), how do they impact the new parents/family?
  - ◆ How is their relationship with their children and grandchildren?
  - ◆ Are they a support for the family?
- **Children**
  - ◆ If an older sibling(s) is present, describe his or her health and social–emotional development.
  - ◆ How is he or she adjusting to the new baby?
  - ◆ Is he or she receiving appropriate attention?

BRIEF FAMILY GENOGRAM

The brief family genogram allows the PCP to diagram and visualize the family relationships. The clinician uses it both to understand the family's problem (current situation) and to discover what they want to accomplish (desired situation). Once a genogram is created, it should be kept in the patient's chart, updated with new information as necessary, and expanded to include other members.

The following 2 case studies illustrate how the clinician can use a brief genogram to help the family understand its particular situation.

CASE STUDY 29.1: THE WELL-CHILD VISIT—THE FAMILY WITH A TODDLER WHOSE PARENTS CANNOT SET LIMITS: USE OF A FAMILY GENOGRAM

During a well-child visit David, a 2-year-old, is out of control. He runs all around the office pulling open drawers, spilling supplies on the floor, and opening and closing the door. His passive, depressed-looking mother angrily and repeatedly, yet ineffectively, tells him to stop but she is unable to enforce her commands. Although the mother does not voice a concern, the clinician raises the subject of the toddler's noncompliance and the need to set limits and suggests a family meeting with both parents.

Family Meeting

During the family meeting, the mother again appears unable to set limits, and David runs all around the room as he had before. The clinician asks the parents if this has happened at home and in public (multiple settings). It has. The father's interactions with David are minimal, but he openly criticizes the mother for not setting limits. The mother's inability to manage David's behavior and the corresponding criticism she receives from her husband leave her feeling depressed and discouraged, which is apparent to the clinician. In response to the clinician's inquiry, the mother reveals that she has felt depressed for several years but that she has not sought help (Figure 29.1, Current Situation).

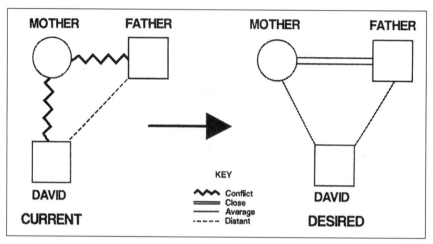

Figure 29.1. Current and desired situations in David's family genogram.

The clinician helps the parents agree on a goal, discusses how they could cooperate with each other, and offers advice on appropriate behavior management techniques. Because the mother's difficulty in setting limits seems associated with her long-standing depression, the father becomes more sympathetic to his wife's struggles. The clinician also suggests a referral to a therapist for the mother, which she accepts (Figure. 29.1, Desired Situation).

Other possible desired situations might include forging a "close" relationship between the father and David and/or between the mother and David or maintaining an "average" relationship between the parents while they both improve their relationship with David.

CASE STUDY 29.2: A 13-YEAR-OLD WHO IS "SAD": USE OF A FAMILY GENOGRAM

First Adolescent Visit

A mother brings in Jimmy, her 13-year-old son, because of his "angry outbursts" at school. Jimmy sits far from his mother with his arms crossed and makes little eye contact with her. This the clinician attributes to "normal teenage behavior." Jimmy's symptoms began approximately 2 months ago when he began slamming doors, kicking walls, and arguing with classmates. His mother feels he is sad because of his father's illness. The clinician carefully interviews Jimmy, who is quiet but cooperative. He has several good friends, and is earning Cs in school. A search for stressors reveals that approximately 3 months ago Jimmy's father had a serious heart attack and was forced into temporary retirement. He is spending his days at home and is participating in a cardiac rehabilitation program. Jimmy is concerned about his father but is glad that his father is getting better. With the loss of the father's income, the mother has taken a full-time job and doesn't get home for dinner until 6:00 pm. This leaves Jimmy and his father home together in the afternoons. Jimmy reports that they watch TV together for an hour and that Jimmy then leaves to join his friends.

The family history reveals no mental illness, but the mother's father had died of a heart attack in midlife when she was a young girl. In a private discussion with the clinician, Jimmy denies sexual activity and alcohol or drug use.

The clinician agrees with the mother's assessment—that Jimmy probably has a good reason to feel sad, but the clinician feels Jimmy is not clinically depressed. He decides against medication for the present but does suggest that the parents try to schedule more family time together. They discuss several ways to do that. Their mood brightens. He schedules a follow-up appointment in 2 weeks.

Second Adolescent Visit

Jimmy and his mother return to the clinic. Jimmy sits far from his mother again and looks sullen. Following the clinician's advice, the mother has tried to schedule more family time, but no one wants it. Jimmy reports, *"Nothing has changed,"* and gives no explanation for his outbursts. The father is continuing his cardiac program and is making slow progress. The mother, who is very worried about Jimmy, urges the clinician to *"do something."* The clinician is also confused. He feels that he is lacking important information about the family, so he asks the mother about scheduling a family meeting, which would also include the father. He explains the purpose of the meeting. The mother agrees and feels that her husband will too.

First Family Meeting

The mother and father sit close together; Jimmy sits some distance from them both (Figure 29.2, Current). The clinician again explains the purpose of the meeting and reviews the history up to this point. He asks Jimmy what he means by *"It's not fair."* Jimmy answers, *"It's not fair that I take the medication. I'm not the one with problems in this family."* When asked what he means by that, he looks at his father but says nothing. The clinician asks the father about his relationship with Jimmy. The father admits that it is *"not as peaceful as you've been told."* The father reveals that when Jimmy comes home from school, he makes many requests of Jimmy (eg, has Jimmy bring him a snack or clean up the house). In the ensuing discussion, the clinician discovers that the father also criticizes Jimmy for not making better grades and for spending so much time with his friends. When Jimmy argues back, the father points to his chest and threatens him by saying, *"If you keep arguing, you'll send me to my grave."* Jimmy, afraid to argue back, instead either retreats to his room or leaves the house, full of guilt and anger. The father also demands that Jimmy not reveal these arguments to the mother and threatens, *"If you do, you'll worry her to death."*

Jimmy feels neglected by his mother because *"she spends every minute with Dad."* Because she is unavailable, he withdraws; their relationship has become distant. Jimmy is angry with his father, and they argue; but Jimmy suppresses his feelings because of his father's threats about his health and the demands to keep the arguments secret from the mother. The relationship between Jimmy and his father is one of conflict.

Jimmy's mother is shocked to hear about this conflict and that both the father and the son have kept their conflict and feelings secret. The clinician asks the family to talk it out at home and to decide how they might improve the family relationships. They agree to try. He makes another appointment.

Second Family Meeting

The family returns in 2 weeks. The members report that they have had a few family talks and that they are feeling a little better. The outbursts have subsided. Further questioning reveals more of the family situation, including the fact that the father is very depressed by his own situation. Compounding his depression is the fact that his own clinician has advised him not to have sexual relations with his wife during cardiac rehabilitation. He wants to resume a normal marital life. Despite urging from his clinician, he refuses to take antidepressant medication because he has heard that it makes you lose your sex drive; he fears that he will lose it forever. He hadn't told his wife that he has stopped taking his medication.

The mother realizes that her memory of her father's death has intensified her concern about her husband so that she has devoted all her time to him, which in turn has isolated Jimmy from her. Jimmy, therefore, is feeling left out by both parents.

The clinician now realizes that Jimmy's anger at school is an expression of the unresolved conflict with his father and of his resentment toward his mother for neglecting him. Many stressors have converged on Jimmy and his parents and have changed their relationships with each other.

Together, the clinician and the parents develop ways to change the family interactions and to meet the family's goals of improving their relationships. The father's goal is to develop a close relationship with Jimmy. Jimmy is not as motivated, but he agrees to cooperate. The father arranges to spend some time with Jimmy each afternoon. They will take walks, play computer games, and occasionally go fishing to develop a better relationship. The father also agrees to undergo a trial of antidepressant medication with the understanding that side effects, if any occur, will not be permanent. If the medication does affect his sexual activity temporarily, his clinician will lower the dose or change the medication. Jimmy and his mother arrange to spend time together each evening. The mother will not devote all of her time to her husband. Furthermore, the family plans to spend more time together in activities, such as reading and going to the library (Figure 29.2, Desired).

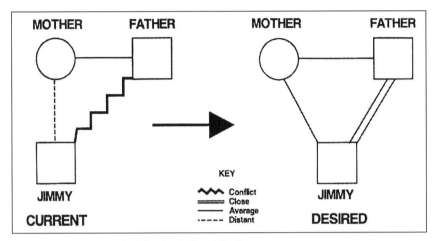

Figure 29.2. Current and desired situations in Jimmy's family genogram.

Third Family Meeting

The family returns in a month. Jimmy and the father have done the things that they had discussed in the previous meeting, and their relationship has improved. The father feels it is close. The father is responding well to medication. His mood is brighter. His rehabilitation is going well. Jimmy and his mother have also followed through on their plans, and their relationship has resumed its "average" status. The family's new interactions are improving the relationships.

Fourth Family Meeting

After another month, they return. As life returns to normal, Jimmy and his father spend less time together. Their relationship has become "average," but it is much better than it had been 5 months ago. The mother and Jimmy have maintained a good relationship. The father's health is improving, and he and his wife have resumed their sexual relationship. He continues to take his medication. The family feels it does not need any more sessions with the clinician, and everyone agrees that this will be the final family meeting.

Chapter 30

Suggestions to Enhance Family Functioning With Case Studies

*F*amilies often come to the pediatric care professional (PCP) for reassurance and guidance. As a PCP the clinician can facilitate the family's own efforts to change its behavior. The clinician can also be directive and make specific suggestions. The family can then modify the clinician's suggested strategy to fit its needs and coping abilities. This chapter describes 6 suggestions (3 are illustrated with case studies) for enhancing family functioning.

Suggested strategies (eg, advice, medication, improved communication) can help if they fit the problem and if the family accepts them. The family can modify a suggested intervention to fit its own style and level of functioning. Suggestions are listed in Box 30.1.

Box 30.1. Suggestions to Enhance Family Functioning
- Feedback: helping parents and children give and receive it (Case Study 30.1)
- Home family meetings
- Special time (Case Study 30.2)
- Resolving family disagreements: natural and logical consequences
- Family rituals and traditions (Case Study 30.3)
- Writing assignments and the compliment box

FEEDBACK: HELPING PARENTS AND CHILDREN BOTH GIVE AND RECEIVE IT

- **Feedback makes parents more effective.** Feedback tells family members how they are doing in the eyes of another. In a behavioral context, it is a way of helping a member understand the impact of his or her behavior on others. Feedback reveals a parent's perception of a child (*"What I hear..."* or *"I'm seeing..."*). Children are more likely to accept feedback (and to respond appropriately) if parents voice it as their perception. Parents often act on their perceptions of a child's behavior, so feedback is important because it gives the child information on how he or she is perceived. Feedback also reveals a parent's perception of himself or herself.

- **Feedback creates dialogue by allowing/encouraging a family member to respond to the feedback.** It gives an individual a chance to explain a behavior, to correct a wrong perception, to appreciate another's feelings, and to change his or her behavior if needed or desired.

- **Feedback is the final step in the teaching and learning loop.** Feedback gives the "learner" information on how well he or she has learned, performed, or behaved. It also enlightens the "teacher" as to how effective he or she is as a teacher, parent, or clinician. Thus the "teacher" and the "learner" both need feedback. In the family meeting, feedback is considered essential; everyone benefits from giving it, receiving it, and responding to it.

CASE STUDY 30.1: A TEENAGED SON NEEDS FEEDBACK FROM HIS PARENTS

The Visit for a Sports Physical

Allen, a 16-year-old adolescent, comes in with his mother for a sports physical examination. The clinician has known Allen for several years, sees him only for occasional school and sports physicals, and knows that he is a good athlete. While examining the boy alone, the clinician inquires about the sports he plays and about his athletic abilities and successes. Allen tells him about his success in baseball. The clinician replies that Allen's parents must be very proud too. Allen's expression and tone of voice suddenly sadden as he states, *"My parents never say anything. They don't come to my games. I wish I knew if they were proud of me."* The clinician asks Allen if he has ever asked his parents to go to the games or has let them know how he feels. Allen replies that he does not ask. The clinician is so impressed by Allen's sadness that he asks if he can share their conversation with Allen's mother. Allen agrees.

Clinician: *I was just talking with Allen. I asked him if I could share our conversation, and he agreed. He wishes you and his father went to his games and feels that he doesn't get recognition or feedback from you and his father about his sports. He wants to know if you're proud of him. He seems pretty sad about this.*

The clinician pauses and remains silent.

Mother: *We are so busy with work. We just started our own business. He knows we're proud. We just don't make a big deal about it.*

Clinician (gently challenging): *How does he know you're proud?*

Mother: *He just does. Besides, feedback is for little kids when they need lots of help. Allen's a young man. He doesn't need it.*

Allen: *How do you know?*

Mother: *Maybe I don't know.*

Clinician (searching for other sources of feedback): *Do you let Allen know how you feel about other things?*

Mother: *If he messes up, he hears about it.*

Clinician (realizing he wasn't making progress with this line of talk, explores instead the family's perception of Allen's sadness): *Allen seems pretty concerned.*

Mother: *You should talk with his dad.*

Clinician (using this comment to suggest a family meeting): *That's a good idea. It would be helpful for all of us to talk. Could you ask your husband?*

First Family Meeting

Engaging the Family

Clinician (explaining the purpose of the meeting): *Thank you for coming in. I know you're busy. I'd like to explain that we're not here to talk about Allen's sadness, although that is what prompted the meeting. Instead I'd like to have a few family talks to help us understand the big picture, which is the apparent reason for his sadness. Your views as parents are invaluable, and together we can find some ways to make things better. How does this sound?*

The family members nod their approval.

Understanding the Family

Mother: *I've been thinking about our last visit. I'd like to see us all tell each other how we are doing but in a way that is helpful and doesn't cause blowups.*

Father: *People need to know when they're screwing up.*

Clinician (bringing the focus back to Allen and what he's doing right): *How about when they're doing well?*

Father: *I can't be running around checking every little thing. Take pride in a job well done.*

Clinician: *Allen, would you like to say something?*

Allen: *Nope. Not now.*

Mother: *There's too much anger.*

Father: *That's right. Some things that Allen does just drive me nuts.*

The clinician looks at Allen, hoping he will engage in a dialogue with his father.

Allen: *Like what?*

Father: *Like not using my tools correctly.*

Allen: *But Dad, you never tell me what I'm doing right or doing wrong. You just blow up.*

The father sits silently.

Mother: *That is what happens. And I do it too. We all do. We forget to tell Allen what he's doing right...like his sports.*

Allen: *What about the tools, Dad?*

Father: *Are you interested?*

Allen: *Sure I am.*

Father: *I always thought you just didn't care about the tools.*

This is a "breakthrough" family interaction in the meeting. The father and son are talking to one another calmly, and they realize they have a common interest. Helping them communicate about the tools could lead to more interactions and understanding that eventually might help resolve the problem that brought them here. At this point, the clinician has decided that the father is the family leader.

Working With the Family

Clinician (keeping the dialogue alive and encouraging the family to develop its own solution): *How could you two get this tool thing going?*

The father starts to address the clinician who asks him to talk to Allen.

Clinician: *Could you look at Allen and talk to him?*

Father (to Allen): *Maybe I could explain how to use the tools, then watch you use them and let you know how you're doing.*

Allen: *You won't get mad at me?*

Father: *Not if you do okay.*

There is a silence. The clinician waits about 15 seconds and then speaks.

Clinician: *How would Allen know he's doing okay?*

Father: *I'd tell him.*

The father appears uncomfortable and unwilling to discuss Allen's feelings. The clinician does not want to alienate the father, so he asks an open-ended question to see if they would follow through with this interaction.

Clinician: *How could you try this during the next week?*

Father (indicating he is not totally sold on this): *It sounds good, but I'm not sure. We'll see how it goes.*

The meeting is ending, and the clinician wants to "model" giving feedback in the form of compliments.

Clinician: *Before you go, I'd like to tell you all that I thought this was a good first meeting. It's just the beginning, but the way you all got right down to business was very impressive.*

Father: *It's no big deal.*

Mother: *See you next week.*

Second Family Meeting

The family reports that Allen and his father have worked together one time and that it went *"okay."*

Clinician (asking them to amplify this success): *Tell me what was okay.*

The father showed Allen how to use the table saw, and he did "pretty well."

Clinician: *Did you tell him?*

Father: *Yeah. He's pretty coordinated.*

Clinician (unable to resist using father's comment as a link to the presenting problem): *After all, he is a good athlete.*

Mother: *I came out and watched them work. It was the first time we had been together enjoyably for some time.*

Clinician (acknowledging another positive interaction): *That must have been pleasant.*

Allen: *When I was cleaning up, we talked about sports.*

Clinician (encouraging more conversation): *What did you talk about?*

Allen: *The Red Sox and my game next week.*

Clinician: *How did that feel?*

Both Allen and his father shrug their shoulders as if to say "okay." The clinician senses that apparently no more can be said about this subject. The rest of the meeting is devoted to discussing a project that Allen and his father will do together.

Third Family Meeting

The family reports that the next session with the tools went well also. The mother joined father and son; after Allen and his father finished the tool project, Allen and his mother talked about sports. The mother declares that she is going to see Allen's next game, but the father expresses no interest. When the clinician asks if the father is letting Allen know how he is doing with the tools, the father says that he isn't telling him but that he feels that Allen is gaining skills by watching and trying.

Father (looking at the clinician): *I don't need feedback on how I am as a dad, and he doesn't need it as a young man.*

The clinician has no response. He determines that, for now, maybe it is enough for this family that they are doing an activity together.

Fourth Family Meeting

At the next visit, the family reports that the tool project has become a regular family event. The mother and Allen have continued their sports talks after the tool project. Each parent has developed an activity, and thus a new relationship, with Allen: the father with the tool project and the mother talking about sports and attending Allen's games. The father, however, is not going to give any more feedback. The family decides that the 4 visits are enough. The clinician asks them for feedback about the effectiveness of the visits. Allen and his mother feel that the meetings have been worthwhile and thank the clinician. The father noncommittally offers a brief "thanks." About a month later, the clinician received a newspaper clipping about Allen and his team. The father had mailed it.

The clinician can help parents and children share feedback with each other. Feedback is more effective under the following conditions:

- **It is specific rather than general.** To tell a child she is "too talkative" is not as effective as saying, *"When we were discussing the birthday party plans, you talked so much I gave up. I felt I couldn't get a word in."*
- **It is descriptive rather than judgmental.** Describing one's own feeling or reaction to another's behavior allows the other person to choose whether to accept it or not and makes a positive response more likely. Sharing one's perception reduces the likelihood of the recipient either responding defensively or ignoring the feedback. Examples of descriptive feedback include, *"I feel happy when I see you sharing with your brother,"* or *"I feel angry when I have to repeat myself over and over about doing homework."*
- **It offers the receiver an alternative or assistance with altering the behavior.** For instance, a parent could say, *"I feel very worried when I see you staying up so late. I am concerned that the lack of sleep makes you feel grumpy. I'd like to discuss how we can help you get to bed earlier."*
- **It takes into account the needs of both the receiver and the giver.** A mother demonstrates this when she says to her son, *"I'd like to talk about getting ready for school. When we argue, you are late for school, I am late for work, and we both feel pretty upset. I'd like to help both of us get out of the house on time."*
- **It is directed toward behavior that the receiver can affect or control.** A child's frustration increases when he or she is reminded of shortcomings over which he or she has little or no influence. Therefore, a parent might

speak to her child in the following way, *"I'd like to help you get along better with your brother. I realize that when you two play sports, he usually wins, and you get upset. I suggest you play board games with him instead of sports all the time. You're good at them, and the two of you could have fun."*

- **It is given at the earliest opportunity after the specified behavior.** Brief, immediate feedback is more effective than delayed, detailed feedback. When a child completes a chore, the parent should acknowledge the accomplishment right away with a positive statement, such as *"Thank you for cleaning your room. I really appreciate it."* Later at dinner or at a family meeting, the parent can give more specific feedback as follows: *"When you cleaned up your room, I was really proud of you. I only asked you once, and you picked up your clothes, put away your toys, and put your books in your pack. That was really great."*

- **The giver considers the receiver's readiness to hear it and accept it.** Feedback should not be given when the giver or receiver is angry. If a child and parent argue about a chore that has not been done, the focus becomes their feelings (or the consequence/punishment) and not the behavior. The parent should wait until the child is more likely to accept the feedback, until the parent is calmer, or until another family member can offer support.

- **It is more effective when support is available.** Feedback often entails giving support. If a child has very poor study habits, he or she usually is disorganized, which often results in losing papers and missing deadlines. The mother can give the child feedback and tell him or her what needs to be done. However, without her support (eg, buying an organizer notebook, restricting TV, and showing the child how to manage time effectively) the child is unable to respond to her feedback even though he or she is willing. In this case, the mother might delay feedback until she is able to provide the support.

HOME FAMILY MEETINGS

The home family meeting is a method of promoting family communication, family and individual tasks, and cooperative behaviors. In the home family meeting every member is encouraged to share his or her thoughts and feelings and to take a legitimate part in family decision-making as determined by the parents. The meeting also allows the family to practice or to repeat at home the behaviors, the cooperation, and the communication of thoughts and feelings that it has already demonstrated in the family meeting in the office or clinic.

When the clinician suggests that the family have a home family meeting, he or she needs to explain the purposes.

Purposes of a Home Family Meeting

The clinician explains the purposes to the family, including the following:

- **To develop cooperative leadership, which gives every member a role, however limited, in family decision-making.** Families need a leader and a hierarchy with the parents at the top. Even though the parents have control, children still need and want to have some say in the decision-making processes. Family conflicts result when the children don't have appropriate input or when they feel they aren't "heard" or appreciated. However, the children must realize that they are not in control. If they are in control, the family hierarchy is seriously unbalanced, and conflicts result. The parents make the decision on how much power the children share. In the meeting, parents share this limited and defined power with the children. Parents should realize that this sharing of power teaches children the values of responsibility and cooperation, but the children must understand and accept that the parents have the final word.

- **To provide a regular, scheduled time for the family members to sit down together, organize the week(s) ahead, and prioritize individual and family activities.** This time allows limited "participatory democracy" and negotiation, prevents schedule conflicts, and safeguards family time from the often crowded schedules of children and parents.

- **To acknowledge and praise the efforts and achievements of the past week(s) (eg, doing a chore or completing a homework assignment).** The meeting can become a time for giving feedback, praising children, and passing out their weekly allowance or earned rewards. Parents also need and should receive acknowledgment and praise. The clinician might encourage the parents to ask the children to make a list of all the things their parents do for them on an occasional basis. The parents should then help the children express their appreciation for everything the parents do. For example, the child might be encouraged to say *"Thank you, Mom, for all the things you have done for me this last week. I didn't realize how much you had done and I love you."*

- **To bring up problems or disagreements that need to be discussed and solved (eg, chores, morning routines, TV viewing, disrespectful behavior, sharing toys).** Although consequences for behavior need to be discussed, the focus of the meeting should not be on disciplinary actions for individuals. The meetings also should not turn into "negative" feedback sessions or scolding lectures. These events should take place at another time in a private setting and on an individual basis that avoids public humiliation.

- **To provide a time that is pleasant and positive for the family.** Members should feel free to discuss things that are working, improving, and going right. Everyone should feel able to talk without fear of being blamed, judged, or cut off. No family member should be scapegoated or humiliated.

- **To inform parents about their children's activities and interests.** Parents often complain that children don't tell them about what they do in school or what their interests are; they feel "left out" and "in the dark." Family meetings provide children the opportunity to be more talkative and to tell parents about their interests. Parents may hear about an activity or game the child enjoys (skating, computer game) and may decide to learn the game or needed skill so that they can participate with their child.

Implementing a Home Family Meeting

The clinician explains how to introduce and begin home family meetings.

- **Introduce meetings at an early age (eg, 4 or 5 years old).** Even if the concept is introduced in adolescence, these meetings succeed because teenagers want to negotiate and share power. All children want attention, which the family meeting provides.
- **Introduce meetings as a positive and appealing family event.** Parents can briefly clarify the purposes (eg, to let everyone share thoughts and feelings, to give praise and rewards, to discuss chores, to plan weekly activities) and also use an inducement that motivates the children (eg, a favorite dessert will be served or allowances will be given).
- **Encourage parents to state that they would like the children's help and to ask them for their thoughts about the family meeting.**
- **Introduce the idea of meetings at a pleasant or neutral time, not in the heat of an argument or after a child has been reprimanded.**
- **Invite the family to participate; don't make the meetings seem like a mandatory event.**

Guidelines for Conducting a Home Family Meeting

The clinician offers these practical tips.

- **Everyone in the home should be invited.**
- **Parents should select a comfortable, quiet place (eg, the living room, the dining room table).**
- **Parents should select the most convenient time (eg, after dinner [with a favorite dessert], Saturday morning, Sunday evening [with a snack]).** The time should be as consistent as possible.
- **Ideally, meetings should be scheduled weekly because that interval provides timely feedback and reinforcement.** A schedule should be posted on a bulletin board or on the refrigerator.
- **During the first meetings, the family should establish time guidelines.** How long should the meeting last? Initially, the meeting should be 20 to 30 minutes in length. Families also need to discuss how long each member is allowed to speak and how much time should be devoted to one topic. To time these once the limits have been decided, parents can use a watch or an egg timer.

- **During the first meetings, the family should determine what issues to discuss.** Chores and general discipline should not dominate meetings and should be discussed early in the meeting. Families should realize that members can share chores but as all family members do not have equal abilities (eg, teenaged son, preschool-aged daughter), chores must also be individualized. Between meetings members can write down topics for future meetings on a piece of paper that they can post on the family bulletin board or on the refrigerator. Younger children can ask parents to include their topic in the next meeting.
- **Keeping a record (minutes) of each meeting (with note taking or a tape recorder) allows the family to keep track of what transpired and minimizes disagreements.** This secretary role should rotate among family members. Agendas should be made and can be posted or handed out (eg, review minutes of the previous meeting, go over the weekly calendar of events, discuss old business, what happened last week, new business, share fun stories, give compliments, and pass out allowances).
- **The leader of the family might consider not chairing the first meeting.** The other parent or an older child might start. This demonstrates that leadership and power are shared and also allows other members to learn leadership skills.
- **Tasks can be assigned at the end of the meeting, and a checklist should be posted in a central location.** Assigning tasks and redefining roles are major goals of the meeting. Expecting each member to be responsible for his or her part is a positive, powerful influence on family functioning.
- **The meetings should always end on a positive note.** Meetings don't always go smoothly, especially in the beginning, but a happy ending encourages the family to continue the meetings. Meetings should end with a family game or activity or with acknowledging effort, giving compliments, or even viewing a favorite TV show or watching a video.
- **If the family wants to cancel a meeting, to shorten or extend a meeting, or to meet at an unscheduled time, parents should be flexible.** If a meeting deteriorates (from arguments, fatigue, lack of interest), it should end—parents should not lecture or scold when family members are angry or tired. The family can discuss what happened the following week and can use the unsuccessful meeting as a lesson. If a member is uncooperative or is feeling ill, he or she should be excused.

SPECIAL TIME

Making time for children is one of the most important things a parent can do. Children want to spend time with their parents, yet parents often discover that finding that time to spend with their children is difficult. Parents want more (and enjoyable) time with their children. Even when parents interact with their children, they often determine the time for the interaction, the amount of time that will be spent on the interaction, and the activity—all of which may detract from the value of the interaction. Special time is one way to fill the deep, constant needs of parents and children for mutual attention and encouragement.

Special time is specifically time together for one child and one parent. The child chooses one parent at a time, and the other parent and children make other arrangements. Parents with 2 or more children should alternate so that each child has time alone with each parent.

Special time provides a form of "time in" for parents and children, an opportunity to spend time with one another, which builds a sense of love, trust, and commitment. It provides predictable, regular, and protected time for the child and parent.

Special time is a prearranged, guaranteed, and uninterrupted time that the parent spends with the child; it is a period of time in which the 2 interact without the parent being judgmental or directive. Each family must decide how often to have special time—daily is ideal. Special time is a time of day in which the parent is unconditionally available to the child. It communicates a commitment to the child and demonstrates by the parent's action that the child is valued and loved.

Special time is suitable for preschoolers, school-aged children, and adolescents.

Purposes of Special Time

The clinician explains the purposes to the family, including the following:

- **It offers children the opportunity to have some input into how parents spend time with them and meet their needs, which makes them feel competent and respected.** Special time defuses a power struggle between parents and children by giving children decision-making power and the self-respect that accompanies that. During special time, the parent might say, *"You're in charge. You pick the activity and I will join you."*
- **Special time can eliminate conflicts.** If a child is pestering the parent to play a game, the parent can respond that he is doing something else at this time, but that *"We can play the game during special time."*
- **Special time allows parents to observe children up close and to focus exclusively on them.** The parent learns much about the child and has many opportunities to praise the child, to encourage him or her, and to express affection.
- **Special time helps parents alleviate their guilt over not spending enough time with their children.** Most parents are busy with work and other responsibilities that leave little time and energy for their children. Special time provides that regular time for children.

Implementing Special Time

The clinician explains how to introduce and begin special time.

- **The parent should suggest the notion of special time at a pleasant or neutral time and should simply ask the child if he or she would be interested in spending time together on a regular basis.**
- **The parent and child select a mutually convenient time of day.** This can vary from weekday to weekend.
- **The child should choose the activity as long as it is within the limits of parental time and financial resources and if it does not violate the dignity or the authority of the parent.** Parents may offer younger children a choice of activities. Suggested activities include reading a story, playing a board game, telling bedtime stories, playing a sport, fixing a broken toy or bike, and going out for a meal. Sharing a musical or artistic activity, going to a museum or library, and cooking a meal are other types of special time. Older children and adolescents may prefer to go shopping, to practice driving the car, or to carry out an activity over several sessions (eg, a time-consuming craft project or a chess game).
- **One of the best opportunities for talking occurs when the parent and the child take car rides so that they are away from the distractions and interruptions of the home.**
- **Generally, interactive activities are preferable, but occasionally, a passive activity (watching TV or a video) is okay.**
- **The parent and child should both decide how much time to spend together based on the parent's ability to keep the commitment.** Starting with short periods is better because then fatigue and boredom are avoided (eg, 15–30 minutes, depending on the age of the child).

Once a schedule has been established, the parent should post it on the refrigerator or in several places (in the bedroom, bathroom, etc). When starting special time, parents often find that it is easy to forget or to cancel.

- **Parents should work hard to keep their promise of special time with the child.**
- **If special time needs to be rescheduled, the parent and the child need to do so together in a democratic manner.**

Guidelines for Special time

The clinician offers these practical tips.

- **Special time should be called by any name that the child chooses (eg, "fun time").**
- **Special time should be given to each child as promised, regardless of behavior or mood.** It is unconditional.

- **If a child is disruptive or uncooperative during special time, the parent has the option to cancel it or to suspend it temporarily until the child settles down.** The parent might want to put the child in time-out for a brief period or to impose another consequence. The parent should decide if the disciplinary action is part of the allotted time or if it is separate.
- **Special time cannot be "saved up" and used to extend the length of the next special time.** Each special time should be for a predetermined amount of time, but sometimes the parent and child may both agree to extend a particular session to finish an activity.
- **Special time should occur without interruption of any kind, unless a true emergency arises.** The other parent or sibling (if able) can help protect special time by answering the phone or helping out with chores.

CASE STUDY 30.2: THE FAMILY WITH CHILDREN WHO ARE "ALWAYS PESTERING US FOR ATTENTION"

Well-Child Visit

During a well-child visit, the 2 children (Jamar, age 5, and Nakesha, age 7) ask endless questions, make repeated requests and attempts to leave the room, and constantly tease each other. The mother's usual responses are, *"Stop that!" "I'll tell you later."* or *"Calm down."* She seems tired and unsure of how to respond and grows increasingly exasperated. She looks at the clinician.

Mother: *You see what's going on. Do you have any suggestions?*

Clinician (acknowledging her feelings): *You seem pretty overwhelmed. Is this what happens at home?*

Mother: *All the time. It has really stressed our family. What can we do?*

Clinician (realizing the need for a family meeting): *I'd like to meet with the family, including your husband. I need you both here* (emphasizing the need for both parents to attend). *I can't offer any sound advice until I learn more about your concern and the family; then we can work on some suggestions.*

Mother: *If I can bring him here, it will be a miracle.*

Clinician: *I can't have the meeting without him. If it helps, I'll schedule a late afternoon meeting.*

First Family Meeting

Engaging and Understanding the Family

The clinician greets the family. She thanks the parents for keeping the appointment and for their punctuality. The father seems a bit tense. The clinician spends a few minutes asking about his work and then explains the purpose of the meeting. The parents agree on their concern—the children are always pestering *"us"* for attention.

The clinician gives the children books and drawing materials and asks them to each draw a picture *"of you doing something with your family."*

Clinician: *First, I'd like to know more about your family routines. Can you describe a typical day?*

The parents both work full time. The children are in after-school programs. Evenings are busy with dinner, homework for Nakesha, baths, TV, and getting ready for bed. The father spends evenings on his computer doing job-related work, but the children *"always want me to play with them."* Weekends are devoted to errands and family activities, but the father often does not participate because he has to *"catch up with work."* This adds to the mother's stress, and the children miss his presence because *"I can't give them the attention they want."*

Mother: *I try to spend time with them, but sometimes I forget; sometimes I have to break my promises because something else comes up.*

Father: *I don't participate as much; but when I do, I must admit that I get frustrated with their endless demands. Then my wife gets upset with me, and the kids get sort of forgotten for the moment.*

Clinician (seeking a goal): *What would you like to see happen?*

Mother: *I'd like us to find a way to give the kids their time and also to have time for my husband and me. Getting everyone organized is challenging at times; sometimes the kids just don't seem to be on the same schedule.*

The clinician explores the family context. The family history is not significant. The maternal grandparents live nearby and love taking care of the kids. The parents are very involved with their church, and the mother teaches Sunday school.

The mother comes from a middle-class background. The father comes from a "working-class poor" background, and his parents divorced early in his life. His mother, who he says was loving, worked 2 jobs, so she was hardly ever home. The father had worked his way through college and states, *"I am very committed to giving my kids a comfortable life. I work very hard, about 60 hours a week at work and at home. I must have gotten that from my mother."*

Clinician: *I see you both care about your kids. Does this leave any time for family life?*

Father: *Not much.*

Mother (angrily): *And not for us as husband and wife.*

Clinician (acknowledging their feelings): *It's hard having a career and being parents and spouses.*

Meanwhile, the children finish their drawings. Jamar's drawing shows his father reading a book to him. Nakesha's drawing shows the family watching

TV. The clinician asks each parent to put a child on his/her lap while the meeting continues.

The clinician compliments the children (reinforcing their good behavior and demonstrating good parenting).

Working With the Family

The clinician hypothesizes that "special time" might decrease the "pestering." It would involve the father, who would spend time with each child, and would give the mother some relief. She decides to use Jamar's drawing as a starting point.

Clinician to father (encouraging one-on-one interaction with Jamar): *Would you like to ask Jamar about his picture?*

Father: *Jamar, you drew a picture of us reading a book. Do you want Daddy to do that some more?*

Jamar smiles and says yes.

Clinician to mother (encouraging mother–daughter communication): *Would you ask Nakesha about her drawing?*

Mother: *Nakesha, tell me about your drawing.*

Nakesha explains that she has a favorite TV program and she wants the family to watch it together.

Clinician (using the family meeting as an example of being "together"): *Like sitting together as you're doing now?*

Nakesha (smiling at her parents): *Yes.*

Clinician (to parents): *Kids are pretty honest, aren't they? What do you think about their wishes?*

The parents agree that the children want some regular time with a parent or doing something together at home, but they still look discouraged. The clinician introduces and explains special time to the parents. She tells them that this could be a way for them to achieve their goal.

Mother (to the father): *If you could be around in the evening or on weekends and not on your computer, we could each give each child that special time.*

Father: *I'm not sure if I can do that. I want to, but I am so consumed with work. But I'll try.*

Concluding the Meeting

The clinician summarizes the meeting by emphasizing the busy lives of the parents, the job demands, their concern for their children, and their willingness to try "special time." Again, she compliments the children for being so well-behaved.

Next Three Family Visits

Effort, Failure, and Disappointment

The family returned for 3 more visits over the next 3 months. They rescheduled 2 of the visits because of the father's work schedule, which resulted in a month-long interval between meetings. This made it difficult for the clinician and the family to work together. In the first month, the parents both carried out special time. They reported that *"the children love it."* The pestering had diminished by about 50%. The mother felt better. Special time had served a useful purpose. When special time worked, they all felt better, which sustained the hope that they still might be happier.

But after that, the father claimed he couldn't do it. His job demands and workaholic style were too demanding. He had broken many promises about meeting the kids for special time, and the kids were very disappointed. The children's pestering increased again, and the parents still had no time for one another.

The clinician had given a directive—that the grandparents take the kids overnight and give the parents an evening together. The parents had done that once, their first date in 6 months.

But now the mother is angry. The stress has strained their marriage. The mother had even considered a trial separation, but now she is willing to work it out, meaning that the husband and wife have decided to get couples counseling from their minister. The clinician acknowledges their persistence and commitment. She likes the family and has great empathy for it but feels that she has done all she can. She lets the parents know that she will continue to be available and supportive to them as their primary care doctor and the family counselor. The parents promise to return, but 6 months later the father is transferred and the clinician never hears from them again.

RESOLVING FAMILY DISAGREEMENTS: NATURAL AND LOGICAL CONSEQUENCES

Natural consequences are normal or natural results of an action. When applied to the parent–child relationship, the parent allows the child to experience the natural consequences of his or her behavior and decisions. Doing this reduces the likelihood of arguments and disagreements between the parent and child or between the parents. For example, if a child breaks his toy on purpose, the result is that he or she has a broken toy that is not replaced by the parents. Children's behavior improves when they experience the consequences of the natural order. Natural consequences are sometimes painful (eg, if a child plays roughly with a cat, the cat scratches; or if a child teases others, he or she is either rejected or teased back). Parents often use natural consequences intuitively (ie, they do not intervene to prevent the consequence).

Sometimes parents cannot allow natural consequences to occur because they are too dangerous, but they can apply logical consequences, which provide the opportunity for parent and child to negotiate choices that fit the nature of the misbehavior.

Logical consequences are extended natural consequences that fit the family's values, time limits, and capabilities. Parents should develop their own logical consequences. They often reduce parental disagreement very effectively, as in the following example. A child rides her bicycle recklessly, and the parents agree that they must impose consequences. However, they disagree on what to do. One wants to spank the child; the other wants to ignore it and let the natural consequence play out—the child might fall off her bicycle and "learn a lesson." However, the child could be seriously hurt, which is unacceptable to the parents. In this case where the parents disagree, the logical consequence (and compromise) could be taking the bicycle away for a week.

If parents do not agree on the use of natural and logical consequences, they and the clinician might use other interventions (eg, other consequences, avoiding high-risk situations).

Purposes of Logical Consequences

The clinician must carefully explain the purposes for using them.

- **They allow children to take more responsibility for their own actions, which enhances their competence and confidence.** The responsibility to change his or her behavior or to face the logical consequence is the child's.
- **They serve as an alternative to parents imposing punishment, a source of parent–child disagreement and conflict.** The "punishment" is the logical consequence of the undesirable behavior. The child experiences the consequence of his or her chosen action.
- **They emphasize actions, not words (eg, threatening, explaining, and persuading).** When parents talk too much, they often become frustrated and angry and overreact (eg, screaming, saying hurtful things or imposing a punishment that is too severe or unrealistic).
- **They can reduce parental disagreement, a major source of family conflict.** When parents differ over punishments, often one parent sides with the child, which in effect forms a coalition with the child and excludes the other parent. Children recognize these patterns and often exploit them, causing considerable family disruption.

Examples of Logical Consequences

In the following examples, the parents explain the consequences before they implement the plan.

- **A child does not put her dirty clothes in the hamper but leaves them scattered around the house.** The mother nags the child to pick them up, but eventually ends up doing it herself. The mother negotiates a plan. If the child puts her clothes in the hamper, the mother will wash them and the child will have clean clothes. If the child does not put her clothes in the hamper, the mother will not wash them and she will not have clean clothes. Of course, the parent must be able to tolerate the child going to school in dirty clothes, and the child must want to wear clean clothes.

- **A teenager refuses to get up promptly in the morning, can't find his books, and often misses the bus.** The parents argue with him and with each other and ultimately drive the boy to school so that he will not be late. They negotiate a plan. If the boy gets up on time and is organized, he catches the bus to school. If he sleeps in, he misses the bus, stays home, and has to figure out his own way to get to school. In this case, the consequence is appropriate if the boy is safe alone and wants to go to school. If he is intentionally avoiding school, the clinician and the family need to investigate the boy's mood and perceptions, the school, and social and learning situations.

- **A child speaks rudely to his parents, who respond with a lot of scolding and threats.** The parents decide to use logical consequences. When another incident occurs, the parents respond, *"This is rude behavior and is not tolerated in our presence. You may speak politely or go to your room."* The child has the choice of being polite or going to his or her room (under escort, if necessary).

- **Siblings fight with each other all day.** The children are given choices. If they play together, they can go to a movie in the evening; if they fight, they miss the movie and spend the evening in their own rooms.

- **A child argues about watching TV beyond his usual time allotment.** The parents negotiate a logical consequence. He can watch his show and then turn off the TV himself. If he does not, TV privileges will be removed for a week.

- **A child refuses to eat her main course at dinner, but she clamors for dessert.** The child can be given a choice: eat the main course first and get dessert second (the logical sequence of a meal) or refuse the main course and get no dessert. If the child has a tantrum, the family may need some guidance on handling that.

Implementing Logical Consequences

The clinician must explain the process for implementing logical consequences.

- **Parents must discuss the choices in advance, in a calm situation, at a neutral time, and not in the heat of an argument.**

- **Parents should provide fair choices that are logical results of the behavior and that fit the family's values and capabilities.**
- **Once the choices are established, the focus shifts to the behavior and talking is minimized.** The child makes the choice and accepts responsibility for his or her behavior.
- **The parents should remain firm and calm.** Maintaining emotional equilibrium and steadfastness is essential parent behavior that strongly influences child behavior.
- **Parents should be flexible.** If a parent has overreacted, become angry, broken an agreement, or imposed a consequence that is too long or harsh, he or she should apologize and renegotiate.

FAMILY RITUALS AND TRADITIONS

Family rituals and traditions give families stability, cohesion, strength, pleasure, and identity. They also provide a sense of connection and belonging to the extended family and the community. Some families have never developed rituals and traditions. Others forget their rituals and traditions when they are working too hard or when they are undergoing a transition (divorce, forming a blended family). The clinician should inquire about family rituals and traditions and should help these families revive or create them.

Traditions like having meals together promote family well-being (eg, greater family cohesion; enhanced coping skills; and reduced risky child behaviors, such as alcohol and tobacco use).

CASE STUDY 30.3: THE FAMILY WITH "NO FAMILY LIFE"

Phone Call

The father of a 12-year-old boy calls because his son Fred seems withdrawn from the family. The clinician schedules a family meeting.

First Family Meeting

Understanding the Family

The clinician briefly socializes with the family and then explains what the family meeting is and how it will work.

Clinician: *I'd like to hear about your concerns.*

Father: *I am concerned about Fred. He seems withdrawn.*

Mother: *He spends lots of time at his friends' homes, but when he is home he's watching TV and on the computer. He's doing well in school, though.*

Clinician (noting that Fred seems somewhat hesitant): *Fred, you might be feeling a little nervous now, and that's normal. But I'd really like to hear from you.*

Fred: *I don't know why we're here.*

The clinician realizes that Fred does not understand the purpose of the meeting. He explains it carefully again. Then he begins to explore the family context.

About a year ago, the father had transferred from California, which removed the family from its life-long home and the extended family members.

Father: *We miss them a lot.*

Clinician (acknowledging the impact on the whole family): *It must be hard on everyone.*

Fred: *We have no family life.*

Clinician (encouraging Fred to talk): *No family life?*

Fred: *Home is boring.*

Clinician (helping the family elaborate): *Can you tell me more?*

Mother: *I think I have an idea. We've never had much of an organized family life. Even before we moved here, we worked all the time, but our relatives were a big part of our lives...holidays, family reunions, occasional picnics.*

Father: *Now we do even less as a family. It's like having three separate lives under one roof, each of us coming and going. We seldom sit down together for meals, and even those are fast.*

After a few minutes of listening to descriptions of the family's lifestyle, the clinician turns to Fred and inquires about his strengths as a way to determine if Fred has some satisfying peer relationships.

Clinician: *Mom said you're doing well in school and have friends.*

Fred: *I really like spending time with my friends.*

Clinician: *What do you do with your friends?*

Fred: *Just hang out with them at their homes. We have fun. More fun than at home.*

Clinician: *Can you explain that a bit more?*

Fred: *We play word games, like hangman or Boggle, sometimes with their parents.*

Clinician: *Do you want that at home?*

Fred: *Yeah.*

Clinician: *Would you consider that your goal—more family life?*

The family clarified family life: regular meal times, family routines, and establishment of some traditions.

Concluding the First Meeting

The clinician summarizes the situation by pointing out the difficulties with the loss of family supports and activities and by reminding the family of its strengths (the members are coping, are attending family meetings, and Fred is doing well in school and has made friends). They will explore some strategies for achieving their goal at the next meeting.

Second Family Meeting

Working With the Family

Clinician: *I have a few ideas in mind, but first what do you think would help?*

Father: *That's why we're here. But our last meeting did help just because we sat and talked together.*

Mother: *We like coming to these meetings, but we know they are only temporary. In a way, they are a routine.*

Clinician (encouraging the members to develop their own solutions): *What could you do to have more family life?*

Father: *Maybe leave my work at the office.*

Clinician: *How could that help?*

Mother: *We could have a regular dinnertime.*

Fred: *With enough time to play Boggle.*

The clinician helps them identify who will be in charge of the 2 tasks: dinner and Boggle. They each describe what they will do. The mother appears to be the family leader, as she leads the talk. The mother will plan 3 meals during the week. The father will get home by 6:00 pm on those days. He will help his wife fix dinner. The mother and Fred will buy a Boggle game, which Fred will be in charge of arranging after dinner. All the family members participate in the planning during the meeting.

Third Family Meeting

The family returns 3 weeks later. Most of the meeting is devoted to discussing what has happened. They have averaged 2 dinners per week. The father just can't do it more. Fred was bitterly disappointed the first time that his father did not come home on time. He cried, retreated to his room, and refused to play Boggle that night. The mother was also upset. The family decided to set the goal for 2 dinners, but Fred had a hard time accepting the change and kept pestering his father. Finally, the mother told Fred that even though it wasn't what he wanted, it was better than before. Maybe later they could try to have 3 dinners a week together.

Clinician: *Do you want to try anything else?*

Mother: *Sunday is the best day for family time.*

Father: *How about church?*

Mother: *We could try it. Fred would see his friends there.*

Clinician: *It's a nice way to get involved with the community. Who's going to be in charge of getting to church?*

Father: *It's my idea.*

Clinician: *Fred, we haven't heard from you.*

Fred: *I want to call my cousins in California.*

The parents agree that calling the relatives every other week would be okay. Fred will be in charge of that task.

Fourth Family Meeting

Three weeks later the family returns. They have attended church weekly. The parents met the parents of Fred's best friend, and they all went out to dinner. Fred had called the relatives in California. The twice weekly family dinners are going well, and Boggle is enjoyed by all. It has been a smooth and pleasant period.

The parents still express some regret that *"life isn't what we'd like"* (they want more dinners at home together), but they are doing okay. The clinician ended the sessions by reminding them of all that they had done. They had established 4 family routines (dinners, Boggle, bi-weekly phone call to the relatives, and attending church). They had also met the parents of Fred's friend and feel that they are more a part of the community.

FAMILY RITUALS AND TRADITIONS (CONTINUED)

Family rituals and traditions create the structure for bringing the family together and leave lasting positive memories.
- **Family activities**
  - **A regular dinnertime**
  - **A video or board game on Sunday evening**
  - **Regular (home) family meetings**
  - **A regular weekly activity (eg, going to the library or a museum, doing errands, working around the house, taking a walk, viewing a favorite weekly TV show, or playing sports)**
  - **A special breakfast on Saturday or Sunday morning (eg, pancakes at home or going to a restaurant)**
  - **Calling, writing, or e-mailing relatives on a regular basis**
- **Other rituals and traditions**
  - **Celebrating holidays and special family events.** Holidays (Thanksgiving, Halloween, the Fourth of July, summer vacations, school holidays) provide an opportunity for the family to come together, to enjoy

family togetherness, to rest, and to celebrate. Celebrating holidays also promotes a sense of family tradition and a feeling of cultural or national identity. It provides a chance to join with other family members and/ or friends.

— **Celebrating special family events (weddings, graduations, birthdays, bar mitzvahs) serves many of the same purposes as celebrating holidays but is more personal and more family-centered.** These celebrations connect family members in a common cause and provide a chance to express affection and support.

— **Participating in spiritual–religious activities.** These traditions and rituals provide families with spiritual and religious strength, a sense of identity, and a connection to the community. Examples include attending weekly services at a religious institution (church, temple, mosque), celebrating religious holidays (Christmas, Hanukkah, Easter, Passover, Ramadan), or practicing a religious or spiritual activity at home (the Friday Sabbath, prayer, meditation).

— **Visiting extended family.** Connecting to the extended family provides a sense of belonging, security, and origin. Examples include visiting or inviting relatives for holidays, birthdays, weddings, and births and taking vacations together.

— **Exploring family history.** Learning about one's family history creates a sense of family identity, history, and pride. Examples include gathering oral family histories from relatives, creating a family timeline, collecting photos and documents for a family album, arranging and/or attending family gatherings, and even visiting family burial sites.

— **Participating in community activities.** Activities in the community offer a connection to the world outside and provide a sense of belonging to something larger, something more than the family. Examples include participating in a school, community, or religious institution activity (bake sales, fund-raising drive, volunteer activities, neighborhood clean-ups, visiting residents in a nursing home) or participating in local sports and recreational activities (eg, those offered through the local YMCA or parks and recreation department).

WRITING ASSIGNMENTS AND THE COMPLIMENT BOX

Writing Assignments

A writing assignment promotes the expression of feelings and thoughts by family members who prefer this kind of expression or who wish to use it from time to time. Many people find that expressing feelings and describing experiences through writing are very therapeutic. Some family members feel more comfortable expressing themselves through writings and drawings than they do vocally. Writing allows the individual to read his or her own mind, to trust the inner feelings, and to improve personal self-image and self-esteem.

Children might write about their parents' divorce, the loss of a friend or relative, a conflict with a friend, the death of a pet, or disappointment over a lost opportunity. They also may want to write about pleasant events, like a family outing, a birthday party, or a personal achievement. Parents might suggest that they write a letter to a family member or friend or that they keep a private journal or diary. Some children prefer writing stories. No matter what form they take, these writing assignments can be private, or they can be shared with an individual or with the whole family.

Clinicians might suggest this activity if they or the parents note that a child is very shy or has difficulty using expressive language (speaking). This also is an excellent technique for children who love to draw.

Parents can introduce the idea of writing assignments in a private conversation with a child or at a family meeting. Parents can also share their own writings as a way to introduce writing assignments.

Children might want to include drawings and photographs with their writing. They should be encouraged to write without worrying about spelling, grammar, or neatness. They can choose any media they want to record their "writings," including by hand, on the computer, or even as a dictation into a tape recorder.

Compliment Box

The purpose of the compliment box is to encourage the expression of compliments and feelings to one another. Clinicians might suggest this if parents and/or children have difficulty with praising each other or with expressing sadness, anger, or happiness. This can also be another way to boost the self-esteem of a child. Family members should write compliments and then deposit them in the box. Each member should write a compliment about another member. The compliments are then shared at dinner, a family meeting, or any other time the family deems appropriate. A member may write a compliment anytime. The idea of a compliment box can be introduced in a family meeting. Compliments reduce blame, negative attitudes, and anger and instill feelings of competence, recognition, appreciation, and love.

Compliments, a form of positive feedback, are a way to acknowledge and recognize another's efforts and achievements. They promote communication. Compliments express affection and increase motivation to do something well and to repeat behaviors that earn praise.

Compliments work for the whole family. Giving compliments is good parenting. They encourage parents to look for what is right and what is working instead of what is wrong. Children should not be the only ones to get compliments. Children should learn to compliment their parents and siblings.

Parents can compliment each other as another way of expressing their appreciation for one another.

Compliments can be verbal (words), nonverbal (smiles, hugs, kisses), and written (notes, letters). Writing assignments and the compliment box are usually short-term solutions to improve family communication and relationships. When they cease to be useful, they are discontinued. If necessary, they can be revived again later.

SECTION F SUMMARY

Assessing and enhancing family functioning includes 3 major categories: (1) observing family activities in the meeting (the family draws a picture together, the child draws a picture, role-playing, hand puppets, and the magic wand), (2) gathering more information about the family with questions and the use of tools (family history, presence of stressors and supports, parenting history, the family life cycle, and family genograms), and (3) offering suggestions to enhance family functioning (feedback, home family meetings, special time, resolving family disagreements, family rituals and traditions, writing assignments and the compliment box).

These suggestions can help any family with its concern and goals. Presently, many American families have a member in the military. Military life, deployment, engagement in battle, being wounded or suffering mental health problems, and re-entry to life at home all have their difficulties. The PCP should be extra mindful that these families are under extra stress.

When considering using any of these strategies, the PCP must always be conscious of the time they consume. These suggestions are most useful after the first interview.

- Observing family activities includes observing family interactions, verbal and nonverbal communication, noting the content of the talk, the "emotional climate" of the family, and noting the "leader" as well as each member's participation. In addition, the PCP can assign tasks such as the family drawing or role-playing to note the family's interactions. These tasks should only be assigned if the PCP feels comfortable and skilled in suggesting them and they seem to "fit" the family's style and level of communication.
- Gathering more information through further interviewing is yet another (and more traditional) way of understanding the family and its circumstances. In addition to the questions mentioned in the detailed description of the family interview (Section D), the PCP can use any of these interviewing strategies, such as family history, presence of stressors and supports, family life cycle, and genogram. Again, questions like the family life cycle and family genogram require extra skill and also can be time-consuming. A complete family assessment may not be necessary; it cannot be and should not be attempted in the first family meeting.

- Suggestions to enhance family functioning are directives. Directives are only useful if the family is ready for them and if they "fit" the family's concern and level of coping. Examples of these techniques are helping parents and children give feedback, use of home family meetings, and exploring family rituals and traditions. Home family meetings are invariably the most useful, most accepted, and most easily implemented of these specific strategies.

Skills Checklist

- Discuss the 3 categories of assessing family functioning. Understand the when, what, and how to determine which strategy to use.
- Provide specific examples of each of the 3 categories.
- Be sure that you, the PCP, practice and feel comfortable with some of these strategies before you use them.
- Discuss how you might have used any of these in the past with your own patients.
- Discuss your own patients/families and consider which of these strategies might be useful in future meetings with particular families.

Suggested Reading

Allmond BW, Tanner JL. *The Family Is the Patient.* 2nd ed. Baltimore, MD: Williams & Wilkins; 1999

Cohen R, Cohler BJ, Weissman SH. *Parenthood: A Psychodynamic Perspective.* New York, NY: Guilford Press; 1984

Coleman WL. *Family-Focused Behavioral Pediatrics.* Philadelphia, PA: Lippincott, Williams and Wilkins; 2001

Coleman WL. Family-focused pediatrics: a primary care family systems approach to psychosocial problems. *Curr Probl Pediatr Adolesc Health Care.* 2002;32:260–305

Coleman WL, Howard BJ. Family-focused behavioral pediatrics: clinical techniques for primary care. *Pediatr Rev.* 1995;16:448–455

DeSalvo L. *Writing as a Way of Healing.* San Francisco, CA: Harper; 1999

Eisenberg ME, Olson RE, Neumark-Sztainer D, Story M, Bearinger LH. Correlations between family meals and psychosocial well-being among adolescents. *Arch Pediatr Adolesc Med.* 2004;158(8):792–796

Franko DL, Thompson D, Affenito SG, Barton BA, Striegel-Moore RH. What mediates the relationship between family meals and adolescent health issues. *Health Psychol.* 2008;27 (2 suppl):S109–S117

Friedman MJ. Posttraumatic stress disorder among military returnees from Afghanistan and Iraq. *Am J Psychiatry.* 2006;163:586–593

Gleason MM. Relationship assessment in clinical practice. *Child Adolesc Psychiatr Clin N Am.* 2009;18(3):581–591

Hahlweg K, Heinrichs N, Kuschel A, et al. Long-term outcome of a randomized universal prevention trial through a positive parenting program: is it worth the effort? *Child Adolesc Psychiatr Ment Health.* 2010;4(1):14–20

Herzer M, Godiwala N, Hommel KA, et al. Family functioning in the context of pediatric chronic conditions. *J Dev Behav Pediatr.* 2010;31:26–34

Hoagwood KE, Cavaleri MA, Serene OS, et al. Family support in children's mental health: a review and synthesis. *Clin Child Fam Psychol Rev.* 2010;13:1–45

Jensen PS, Martin D, Watanabe H. Children's response to parental separation during operation desert storm. *J Am Acad Child Adolesc Psychiatry.* 1996;35:433–431

Josephson AM. Practice parameter for the assessment of the family. *J Am Acad Child Adolesc Psychiatry.* 2007;46:922–937

LaRosa AC, Glascoe FP, Marcias MM. Parental depressive symptoms relationship to child development, parenting, health and results on parent-reported screening tools. *J Pediatr.* 2009;155(1):124–128

Mansfield AJ, Kaufman JS, Marshall SW, et al. Deployment and the use of mental health services among US army wives. *N Engl J Med.* 2010;362(2):101–109

Tanner JL. Separation, divorce, and remarriage. In: Carey WB, Crocker AC, Coleman WL, Elias E, Feldman HM, eds. *Developmental-Behavioral Pediatrics.* 4th ed. Philadelphia, PA: Elsevier; 2009:125–134

Wilson S, Durbin CE. Effect of paternal depression on fathers' parenting behaviors: a meta-analytic review. *Clin Psychol Rev.* 2010;30(2):167–180

Wissow LS, Gadomski A, Roter D. Improving child and parent mental health in primary care: a cluster-randomized trial of communication skills training. *Pediatrics.* 2008;121(2):266–275

Special Topics

Chapter 31

Making a Mental Health Referral With Case Study

PURPOSE

Clinicians frequently encounter problems that exceed their capabilities and therefore require a referral to an agency or another professional (hereafter called mental health professionals). Making a mental health referral, an important part of family counseling, requires skill and sensitivity. This chapter describes the elements of the referral process, including gaining the family's trust, learning about benefits of mental health insurance plans, giving descriptions of various mental health professionals, working with mental health professionals, and conducting follow-up visits.

ELEMENTS OF THE REFERRAL PROCESS

The clinician often encounters psychosocial problems that require referral to a mental health professional. The referral might be for the child (eg, depression), a parent (eg, alcoholism), the parents (eg, marital conflict), and/or the entire family (eg, relationship/communication problems).

The referral process is a multi-element process, the components of which are listed in Box 31.1.

Box 31.1. Elements of the Referral Process

- Gain the family's trust
- Know the mental health professionals in the community, and develop a relationship with them so that referrals are more personalized and specific
- Know when to refer
- Know which problems to refer
- Discuss the referral with the family
- Mental health benefits of the health plan and description of various professionals: what the family needs to know
- When the clinician chooses the mental health professional: what the clinician needs to know
- The clinician and the mental health professional: working together
- Follow-up visits: what happens to the child and family after the referral
- When a referral fails
- Locate mental health professionals

CASE STUDY 31.1: THE FAMILY WITH A CHILD WITH ATTENTION-DEFICIT/HYPERACTIVITY DISORDER AND PARENTS WHO ARE EXPERIENCING MARITAL CONFLICT

First Child Visit

The mother of Joey, a 10-year-old boy who was diagnosed with attention-deficit/hyperactivity disorder (ADHD) 2 years before, makes an appointment because the *"ADHD is coming back."* Joey had been doing well in school and had been relating well to his peers. Initially he responded well to medication, but about 4 months ago he became irritable and hyperactive. The clinician reviews the situation, but neither the teacher nor Joey and his mother identify any recent stresses. The clinician increases Joey's daily medication dose.

Next 3 Child Visits

During 3 more visits over a 2-month period, Joey's symptoms do not improve. The clinician focuses on Joey and his symptoms and prescribes different medications and combinations of various medications. Each attempt fails to alleviate the symptoms. The mother becomes increasingly frustrated (*"the medicine isn't working"*). Joey appears to have little insight into his difficulties as he responds to most questions with, *"I don't know."* At the fourth visit, the father joins the mother and Joey because he says that he is very worried because Joey's *"ADHD is really stressing our family life."* The father reports that Joey has been sent to the principal's office 2 times for defiant behavior. The father appears defeated (*"I don't know what to do."*), and Joey refuses to talk about it.

Clinician (seeking to understand the impact on the family): *How are you responding?*

Mother: *I'm upset with everyone.*

Clinician (clarifying): *Everyone?*

Mother (not answering the question): *There's just a lot of strain.*

Her eyes well up with tears.

Clinician (acknowledging her feelings and exploring the family's coping ability): *Sometimes when a child has a problem, the family has a hard time coping, which makes things even more difficult.*

Father: *We're having a hard time.*

At this point, the father and Joey exchange glances.

The clinician is confused and realizes that he needs to know more about the family (eg, family history, recent changes, and the parents' relationship).

Clinician: *It's very apparent that it's been hard, and I appreciate your openness. Our time is almost up, but I'd like to make our next meeting a family meeting.*

He explains the purpose of the meeting.

The parents exchange glances. Joey looks back and forth from parent to parent.

Mother (expressing doubt about a family meeting): *I'm not sure if that would be helpful.*

Clinician (gently confronting and clarifying): *Can I ask what you mean?*

The father answers for her. He states that they will think about it. He then asks if they would have some time alone with the clinician. The clinician answers affirmatively.

GAINING THE FAMILY'S TRUST

When the family trusts the clinician, they are more likely to reveal important information and to accept a referral. The clinician gains the family's trust, which is the basis of a good clinician–family relationship, by respecting the family's stated concerns, joining with all the members, and working with them in a professional and supportive manner. Two potential clinician–family relationship problems hinder the referral process. If the relationship is one of "disengagement" (distant, remote), the family might interpret the clinician's referral as a sign of disinterest or of disdain for the family. The clinician can prevent this by taking time to get to know the family, supporting the parents and the child, and acknowledging every member's feelings. If the clinician–family relationship is one of "enmeshment" (overly involved, very attached), the family may interpret the referral as a sign of rejection, disappointment, and loss. Clinicians can prevent this by maintaining a family systems perspective, by monitoring their own behavior, and by examining feelings that the family evokes in them. See Section C (Chapter 14) for further discussion.

KNOWING WHEN TO REFER

Clinicians often make a referral under the following circumstances:
- When the family is a friend or social contact of the clinician
- When the clinician and family agree about the urgency of a situation (eg, an acute crisis)
- When the presenting problem falls outside of the clinician's abilities (eg, alcoholism)
- When the family requests a referral
- When the real problem or the hidden agenda is revealed after several visits, and it exceeds the clinician's skills (eg, domestic violence)
- When the clinician has worked at length with the family, but the numerous interventions have failed (The clinician is confused, and the family is frustrated. The clinician can assume that after 3 to 4 visits if the family is not progressing to everyone's satisfaction, the clinician should make a referral.)

KNOWING WHICH PROBLEMS TO REFER

Determining which problems to refer can be difficult if the family has a hidden agenda or a family secret or if the clinician focuses too exclusively on the symptom and/or fails to explore the family context.

Nature of the Problem

The clinician must first decide if the nature of the problem falls within his or her own interest or expertise. Some clinicians have interests and skills in a broad range of problems (eg, communication problems, mood disorders in children, parental disagreements, and sibling rivalry). Others have a narrow range of skills and interests (eg, ADHD in children). Some clinicians prefer to work with toddlers and families; others prefer to work with adolescents and families.

Clinicians working at the level of family involvement (assessing the concern and the solution within the family context) should refer the family if the family has not responded to their efforts. For example, if the clinician has attempted to work with the family in reducing tension and arguments and has failed, the family should be referred. See Chapters 2 and 5, for more discussion.

Severity of the Problem

The clinician should assess or estimate the level of severity of a problem when considering a referral. Factors that influence the clinician's perception of the problem or that indicate severity include the following: disproportionate parental worry, the affected domains of function of both the child and the family, and a preponderance of risk factors.

- **Parental worry can influence the clinician's perception of the problem.** Some parents may be too worried about a problem; this worry stems from their anxiety, overprotectiveness, or unrealistic expectations for themselves and the child. They may exaggerate, or even exacerbate, the symptoms and insist on unnecessary tests or treatments. The parents' anxiety affects the clinician, causing him or her to overestimate the severity so that he or she feels compelled to make a referral. On the other hand, some parents do not worry enough about a problem. They may be in denial, unaware of the implications of the problem, or distracted by other life issues. Their attitude may lull the clinician into agreeing with their perception of the problem; as a result, the clinician underestimates the severity of the child's problem. The clinician must determine the appropriateness of the parents' worry and help them adjust their level of concern to "fit" the problem. Once the parents' level of concern is appropriate for the problem, they are more likely to accept the clinician's diagnosis and to work with him or her.

- **Affected domains of function are those areas of the child's and family's functioning that are influenced by the problems.** The child's depression may be severe enough to affect his or her school learning and peer interactions. The family hierarchy may break down so that boundaries become diffuse. A sibling may be ignored, or the marriage may be strained. The pervasiveness (number of affected domains or sites) and the functional impairment (severity of the impact) help the clinician determine the severity of the problem and the level of help needed.

- **Assessing both the risk and protective factors helps the clinician consider the overall level of severity.** Risk factors exert a destabilizing or negative influence on the child and/or family; protective factors exert a stabilizing or positive influence. Assessing these factors helps the clinician determine the level of severity. The clinician might treat a child with depression (instead of referring him or her) and suggest a referral for the child's father to Alcoholics Anonymous for his drinking problem. The clinician might refer a child with bipolar illness in a multi-problem family to a child psychiatrist and a social worker. Protective factors should be recognized and nurtured (eg, a family should be encouraged to reach out to its extended family for support; a family's willingness to meet and talk should be nurtured through office visits).

  Child risk factors can include medical or emotional illness, difficult temperament, and learning problems. Family risk factors include teenage parents, divorced/single parent, unemployment, poverty, lack of transportation, inadequate housing, homelessness, marital conflict, parental depression, and alcoholism or drug abuse.

Protective child–family factors incorporate the child's good medical health; success in school; an intact family; financial security; and/or being involved with the local church, temple, or mosque. Community protective factors include access to medical and mental health resources, affordable housing, a crime-free neighborhood, the presence of friends, and recreational facilities. Protective factors provide a buffer for the child and family and reduce the impact of risk factors.

Discussing the Referral With the Family

After the clinician decides to refer, he or she needs to consider the following issues: when to discuss the referral in the meeting; how to help the family understand the problem and need for a referral; the family's past experiences with mental health services, if any; and how to explain the referral to the family.

- **When to discuss the referral in the meeting.** The idea of referral should be voiced early enough in the family meeting so that sufficient time remains to review past interventions, explain the reasons, describe the referral process, and answer questions. If too little time is left, the clinician should schedule another meeting. Sometimes the idea of a referral arises during a parent–child visit for a behavioral problem that initially seems simple and mild. The clinician must decide whether to discuss a referral then or to schedule a family meeting instead. The family meeting is preferable for the following reasons:
  - It provides additional information that helps the clinician select the most appropriate mental health professional.
  - The family should discuss it (and usually wants to) and should decide as a family with the clinician present.
  - The family leader must approve the referral.

CASE STUDY 31.1 (CONTINUED)

Family Meeting

During the pre-interview phase before the family meeting, the clinician considers the following. Joey has been doing well until 4 months ago. No obvious stresses have been identified, and medication trials have failed to improve the symptoms of his ADHD. Joey is doing worse, and at the last visit the parents seemed discouraged. When the mother mentioned the family strain, she was especially sad. The clinician senses that the problem exceeds his capabilities. He thinks a referral might be needed, but he is not sure what kind of referral is necessary. He needs more information to help him understand the problem within a family context. During the family meeting he plans to

1. Review Joey's situation, focusing first on Joey (still the identified patient), and then allow the family to respond.
2. Explore family relationships, and let the family respond.
3. Suggest an appropriate referral.

Clinician (after greeting the family): *We're meeting because you want to see Joey doing better. Meeting as a family helps everyone understand the problem better and find appropriate solutions. Let me briefly review the situation.* [After he reviews it] *Let me hear from you. What are your thoughts and reactions?*

The parents state that they are mystified and that they hope that the clinician can help. They have spoken with Joey's teacher, who is supportive but who is also confused.

Clinician (getting Joey involved): *Joey, what would you like to say? We need to hear from you too.*

Joey: *I want things to be good again.*

Clinician (acknowledging Joey's feelings): *Joey, I know this has been hard on you and I appreciate you being here.*

Joey looks down and is silent.

Clinician (seeking clarification and more information): *What do you mean by "be good again?"*

Joey continues to look down and does not respond.

Clinician (exploring the parents' perceptions): *This must be hard on you too. What do you think Joey means?*

Parents: *We think he wants to end his ADHD problems.*

Clinician (exploring the parents' coping abilities): *How do you respond to Joey's problems?*

The parents do not punish him for the problems at school, and they both give him extra attention at home.

Clinician (using the mother's comment in the previous visit about "strain" to expand the inquiry): *At our last meeting you mentioned "lots of strain" and seemed very sad.*

The clinician purposefully states this in an open-ended manner without asking a specific question. He pauses and waits.

The mother starts to say something, but she looks at Joey and hesitates.

Clinician (deciding that he needs to speak with the parents only and remembering the father's request for "time alone"): *I'd like to excuse Joey for a few minutes so we can talk. Joey, you can wait in the playroom.*

When they are alone, the clinician sits silently to let the parents compose their thoughts and speak first. They sit silently for 15 to 20 seconds, staring at the floor and exchanging glances. Neither seems willing to talk. The clinician decides to begin by using an indirect opening—focusing on Joey—not on the parents or their relationship, as they seem hesitant and uncertain.

Clinician: *Have there been any stresses or strains that might be influencing Joey?*

The parents explain that they have been experiencing marital tension for almost a year. Several months ago, it escalated to heated arguments. Although they waited until Joey had gone to bed, they were sure that he heard them yelling and crying but they did not know how to tell him or even if they should. They have not told anyone (teacher, relatives, friends) about their marital problems.

Clinician (probing the parents' perception of a possible link between their problems and Joey's problems): *Do you think that the marital tension affects Joey and that his problem is not just ADHD?*

Mother: *It must.*

Father: *Maybe.*

- **The family's experience with referrals.** The clinician should inquire about the family's past experience with referrals (if it has had any and if those referrals were successful) and about preconceived fears or beliefs about mental health professionals. Thus informed, the clinician can avoid making the same referral or making it in a way that has failed or has been rejected by the family in the past. The clinician tailors the referral to produce the best match with the family's needs and beliefs. Below are several questions the clinician can use to make the appropriate determination.
  — *"In the past have you or any family member been referred to a counselor or mental health professional? If yes, what was the problem?"*
  — *"Who made the referral?"*
  — *"Did you understand the reason for the referral?"*
  — *"Did you keep the appointment? If not, what happened?"*
  — *"Who (what type of counselor) did you see?"*
  — *"What happened? What was the counselor's approach?"*
  — *"Was it helpful? If yes, why? If no, why not?"*

CASE STUDY 31.1 (CONTINUED)

When actually suggesting a referral, the clinician frames it as something that other people experience as well.

Clinician (introducing the idea of a referral): *Every couple experiences problems in their marriage. Sometimes they get to a point where they need some professional help. This is especially true when the marital problems affect the children.*

The clinician pauses to give Joey's parents a chance to respond. They nod slightly and look at each other.

Clinician (after about 15 seconds of silence): *Have you ever seen anyone or considered getting help?*

The father (revealing an experience that influenced his attitude) replies that friends of theirs had gone to a marriage counselor but that the husband felt he was being blamed for everything, so after 2 visits he stopped going. His friends' experience makes him doubt the usefulness of marital counseling.

The mother (revealing another influence) replies that her mother tells her to *"just hang in there,"* which she has tried but it isn't working.

- **How to explain the referral.** If the clinician has not done so yet, he or she should now briefly review the problem and any attempted interventions and outcomes. The family is more likely to accept a referral if the clinician takes the following actions:
  — Makes sure that family members understand the problem and its impact on family functioning.
  — Helps them understand that a referral is necessary.
  — Clearly explains the potential benefits of a referral to the parents and the child.
  — Has personal or specific information about the mental health professional.
  — Does not imply that he or she is trying to "get rid of" the family.
  — Provides follow-up visits with the family.

CASE STUDY 31.1 (CONTINUED)

The clinician summarizes the situation and reviews the apparent relationship between the marital problems and Joey's feelings/behavior.

Clinician: *You have shared that you've had marriage problems for a year, but you've hesitated to seek help. You agree that the marriage problems are affecting Joey; his problems began occurring about the same time your problems were intensifying. He is probably feeling sad and anxious that you might separate or divorce. Sometimes children blame themselves for their parents' problems, which only adds to their worry. At other times they are angry with their parents. Joey's behaviors and moods at school may be an expression of all of these feelings.*

WHEN PARENTS AND THE CLINICIAN DISAGREE

Parents may disagree that "their problem" is affecting "the child's problem." The clinician should not force his or her viewpoint on the parents. They will become defensive. Instead, the clinician should propose that a combination of child factors (temperament, neurodevelopmental status) and family–social factors may explain the "child's problem." Parents sometimes need time to think about the referral or to speak with friends or relatives.

Father: *I hadn't realized how worried Joey was about us. I just thought he was worried about his ADHD and his school behavior.*

Mother: *I feel so bad that we have waited so long.*

Clinician (emphasizing the need to attend to the marital problem): *It sounds to me like you both agree that resolving the marital problem is important.*

> They nod.

Clinician (mentioning the referral very openly and directly): *Would you like me to suggest a counselor, or do you want to look around and see who is on your health plan?*

> The parents decide to find a counselor who is on their health plan.
>
> The clinician should suggest the referral in a confident, supportive, and directive manner.

Clinician: *I know you feel hesitant about seeing a marriage counselor, but I also feel very strongly that it would be helpful.*

> The parents nod.

Clinician (anticipating a common occurrence and planning an alternative strategy): *If that counselor is not the right fit for you, I can help you find another.*

> The parents nod silently.

Clinician (letting the family know that he wants to follow it during/after the referral process): *We will continue the family meetings until Joey is doing better.*

MAKING A REFERRAL

The clinician should give the family names and phone numbers of mental health professionals whom he or she can recommend with confidence.

Some families do better if the clinician calls to make the appointment while the family is in the office.

Mental Health Benefits of the Health Plan and Descriptions of Various Professionals: What the Family Needs to Know

The clinician can recommend/choose a mental health professional for the child/family, or the family can choose its own; sometimes the family's choices are limited to those endorsed by its health plan. Regardless of who chooses the mental health professional, the family needs to know the mental health benefits of its health plan. The clinician might have this information available so that he or she can share it with the family, or the family can obtain it from its health plan (Box 31.2).

> **Box 31.2. Mental Health Benefits of the Health Plan: What the Family Needs to Know**
>
> - What mental health services are covered by the family's insurance policies, health maintenance organization, or preferred provider organization?
> - Is the recommended professional approved as a provider by the family's insurance company or organization?
> - What percentage of the professional's fees is covered by the policy?
> - Is there a limit on the number of visits per year? Over the life of the policy?
> - Does the policy cover psychological tests and evaluations?
> - Does the policy cover psychotherapy (talk therapy) and/or medications?
> - Does the family need to get a referral first from its primary care provider?
> - What happens if the entire family or certain members do not like the recommended professional?
> - What happens if the family wishes to use a professional from outside the network of approved providers?

When families inquire about their mental health benefits, they are sometimes given a list of professionals by their health plans. Adherence may be better if the clinician gives only one name of a mental health professional, if possible. Sometimes families are unclear about the differences (eg, training or the field of expertise) among various professionals. Below are descriptions of various professionals who can provide mental health services/counseling.

- **Psychiatrist (MD or DO).** This individual has formal training in adult psychiatry. A child and adolescent psychiatrist has extra training (usually a 2-year fellowship working with children or adolescents). Some psychiatrists practice individual, marital, and family therapy. Others may specialize in other areas (eg, substance abuse). Psychiatrists can prescribe medications.
- **Behavioral–developmental pediatrician (MD or DO).** This individual has 3 years of general pediatric training and extra training (a 2- to 3-year fellowship) in behavioral pediatrics and/or child development. Fellowships vary greatly in their emphasis—some focus on infants and young children with developmental disabilities and others focus on all ages and a broad range of problems. Pediatricians can prescribe medications.
- **Family physician (MD or DO).** This practitioner has 3 years of general family medicine training and, possibly, extra training in family counseling/ therapy. Family physicians can prescribe medications.

- **Clinical psychologist (a counselor with a master's degree [MA] or doctoral degree in psychology [PsyD or PhD] or education [EdD]).** These individuals can provide clinical services that include both diagnosis/assessment (eg, mental health, cognitive ability, academic achievement) and therapy (eg, individual, group, marital, or family). Those with a doctoral degree have completed graduate school with the accompanying practicum, a dissertation, and a clinical internship. The psychologist should be listed in the National Register of Health Services Providers and licensed by the state. Psychologists cannot prescribe medications.
- **Social worker (a counselor with a bachelor's degree [BSW], master's degree [MSW], or doctoral degree [DSW or PhD]).** Social workers are accredited by the Academy of Certified Social Workers if they have a master's degree from an accredited school of social work, have completed 2 years of supervised work, and have passed a written examination. Social workers have a wide range of skills and interests (eg, assessing the family–social environment) and providing counseling (eg, individual, family). The National Association of Social Workers keeps a national register of clinical social workers. Social workers cannot prescribe medication, and the family should be aware of this.
- **Psychiatric nurse (registered nurse [RN]); psychiatric nurse practitioner.** This individual has completed a 4-year nursing program and an 18- to 24-month master's program (academic and clinical work with supervision) in psychiatric training focused on children, adolescents, and families. After passing a national examination, psychiatric nurses are certified by the American Nurses Association. They cannot prescribe medications.
- **Marital and family therapist (master's degree [MA] or doctoral [PhD or MD]).** In addition to the advanced degree, these individuals have completed many hours of supervised training in marital and family therapy. Only MDs can prescribe medication, and the family should be notified of this.

When the Clinician Chooses the Mental Health Professional: What the Clinician Needs to Know

If the clinician recommends a specific mental health professional, knowing something about this individual (style and approach) to provide a good "fit" between the counselor and the client/patient is helpful. The clinician can learn about local mental health professionals in several ways: talking to them on the phone; meeting them for lunch; and inviting them to give talks at grand rounds, office practice meetings, and state medical society meetings. Reading their reports and soliciting feedback from those who have worked with these specialists (colleagues, families, and school counselors) can give additional insight. Local and state mental health associations provide some background information. Below are some helpful questions the clinician should consider.

- What are the modalities of treatment (eg, medication, behavior modification, individual and/or family therapy)?
- How available is the specialist to the family (eg, does he/she return phone calls)?
- Does the specialist accept low-income families?

REFERRALS AND THE HEALTH PLAN

In the era of managed care, the clinician has less control over who the child, parent(s), or family may see on a referral basis, but the clinician can learn about the approved mental health professionals and may be able to direct the family to a particular individual.

- How long will the family have to wait to get an appointment?
- Are appointment times flexible and convenient for the family?
- Where is the specialist's office located? How convenient is it for the family?

CLINICIAN AND THE MENTAL HEALTH PROFESSIONAL: WORKING TOGETHER

The clinician and the mental health professional often collaborate in several ways, as listed below.

- The mental health professional provides specialized services (eg, marital therapy), and the clinician provides primary care for the family (eg, counseling and individual interventions for the child).
- The mental health professional treats the child/family for a specified number of visits, and then the clinician continues the treatment.
- The mental health professional serves as an occasional consultant to the clinician, and the clinician provides all of the treatment.

The clinician and the mental health professional should develop a working relationship that provides the best care for the child and family.

Elements of a Good Working Relationship Between the Clinician and Mental Health Professional

Communicating the Specific Purpose of the Referral to the Mental Health Professional

When making the referral, the clinician should clearly communicate the purpose of the referral (eg, refer Joey to a child psychologist or psychiatrist to evaluate Joey's situational sadness/anxiety and recommend treatment [medication, individual therapy with a mental health professional, or continued family counseling with the clinician]).

Defining the Responsibilities of the Clinician and Mental Health Professional

When the mental health professional and the clinician are both physicians, they must decide who is prescribing the medication. If a child psychiatrist is seeing a child with severe psychiatric illness, the psychiatrist should prescribe the medication and the clinician should provide family counseling and well-child care. The family should be informed so they know who to call for help or advice for a particular problem.

When the mental health professional is not a physician providing individual child therapy and the clinician is prescribing medication, they need to define their roles and respect each other's expertise. If the parents have a question about medication, they should consult the clinician. If they have a question about therapy, they should first consult the mental health professional.

Exchanging Information Between the Clinician and the Mental Health Professional

The clinician and the mental health professional need to decide what information to exchange with each other. This information might include detailed background information at the time of referral, their hypotheses, detailed or general summaries of each visit, a summary every few months or only at the end of treatment, and/or notification if the family has not kept its appointments. The clinician and the mental health professional can decide on the best way to communicate (eg, office and home phone, e-mail, or dictated notes).

Clinician–Specialist Relationship

Some families may not want the clinician to know everything they share with the mental health professional. Some specialists prefer not to share information with the clinician even though the clinician and family want to share it. When these issues arise, the clinician, the family, and the mental health professional should resolve them expeditiously. Get permission from the family to share information with the specialist.

FOLLOW-UP VISITS: WHAT HAPPENS TO THE CHILD/FAMILY AFTER THE REFERRAL?

Follow-up visits are an integral part of ongoing child and family care. A referral does not mean that the clinician is abandoning the family or is relinquishing his or her role as a care provider or advocate for the family.

After the referral, the clinician should schedule a follow-up visit to assess the family's progress and its satisfaction with the mental health professional. Knowing the clinician is still interested, involved, and available comforts the family. Follow-up visits enable the clinician to reevaluate the child and the family, to interpret new information, and to incorporate these data into the profile of the family (eg, adding information to the genogram).

Follow-up With the Specialist

The clinician should ask the mental health professional to notify him or her if the family does not keep the initial appointment.

When a Referral Fails

The clinician may learn of an unsuccessful referral with a communication from the mental health professional, through a follow-up visit, or by a phone call to the family.

When a referral fails, the clinician can take the following actions:

- Phone the family or schedule a meeting to discuss why the family members think the referral did not work with the mental health professional if they feel comfortable doing so. A misunderstanding between the family and the mental health professional might be cleared up, and the family might resume treatment.
- Remind the family that sometimes 1 or 2 visits with the mental health professional are needed to clarify expectations and to establish a comfortable relationship.
- Obtain information from the mental health professional if the family consents (signs a consent form). The clinician might share the information with the family.
- Help the family find another mental health professional if it is still motivated.
- Address other specific problems (eg, helping the family find an affordable mental health professional).
- Reassess the family's problems in light of new information, and/or continue to explore the family context to make a more appropriate referral if it is still interested.
- Maintain contact with the family if it refuses a second referral; if and when the problem worsens, the family may accept the referral.
- Continue to see the family, and help it (within the clinician's capabilities). The family may or may not opt to try another referral.

Family Refusal of the Referral

When a family refuses a referral, the clinician should continue to see the family, understand its reason for the refusal, and help it appreciate the benefits of the referral. The clinician can also consult the mental health professional for advice on how to continue to support the family while attempting to convince it to accept another referral.

LOCATING MENTAL HEALTH PROFESSIONALS

The clinician can locate mental health professionals in the community and state in several of the following ways:

- Ask colleagues.
- Contact state and local mental health associations.
- Call universities (eg, school of social work, department of psychology).
- Call academic medical centers (eg, departments of psychiatry, pediatrics, family medicine, and nursing).
- Contact private mental health professionals.
- The clinician can also obtain names and addresses of local or state mental health professionals through lists of national organizations.

Professional Organizations

American Academy of Child and Adolescent Psychiatry
3615 Wisconsin Ave NW
Washington, DC 20016-3007
Phone: 202/966-7300
Web site: www.aacap.org

American Association for Marriage and Family Therapy
112 S Alfred St
Alexandria, VA 22314
Phone: 703/838-9808
Web site: www.aamft.org

American Psychiatric Association
1000 Wilson Blvd, Suite 1825
Arlington, VA 22209
Phone: 888/357-7924
Web site: www.psych.org

American Psychological Association
750 First St NE
Washington, DC 20002-4242
Phone: 202/336-5500
Web site: www.apa.org

National Association of Social Workers
750 First St NE, Suite 700
Washington, DC 20002-4241
Phone: 202/408-8600
Web site: www.naswdc.org

General Organizations

Substance Abuse and Mental Health Services Administration
1 Choke Cherry Rd
Rockville, MD 20857
Phone: 800/789-2647
Web site: www.mentalhealth.org

National Alliance on Mental Illness
3803 N Fairfax Dr, Suite 100
Arlington, VA 22203
Phone: 800/950-6264 or 703/524-7600
Web site: www.nami.org

Mental Health America
2000 N Beauregard St, 6th Floor
Alexandria, VA 22311
Phone: 800/969-6642 or 703/684-7722
Web site: www.nmha.org

SUMMARY

Making a mental health referral is one of the clinician's most important jobs. The clinician is more likely to make a successful referral if it is done in an organized, sensitive, and supportive manner. The referral process includes several aspects.

- Gaining the family's trust
- Knowing when and what problems to refer
- Discussing the referral with the family
- Helping parents know the mental health benefits of their health plans
- Knowing and locating the mental health professionals in the community
- Collaborating with the specialist
- Helping the family deal with unsuccessful referrals

Skills Checklist

- The pediatric care professional (PCP) should be very clear and honest with himself or herself about his or her clinical skills and know what kinds of families or aspects of family problems necessitate a referral.
- The PCP should discuss the following aspects of making a referral:
  — Gaining the family's trust
  — Knowing when and what problems to refer
  — Discussing the referral with the family
  — Helping parents know the mental health benefits of their health plans
  — Knowing and locating the mental health professionals in the community
  — Collaborating with the specialist
  — Helping the family deal with unsuccessful referrals

SUGGESTED READING

Bailey D, Garrada ME. Referral to child psychiatry: parent and doctor motives and expectations. *J Child Psychol Psychiatr* 1989;30:449–458

Breitenstein SM, Hill C, Gross D. Understanding disruptive behavior problems in preschool children. *J Pediatr Nurs.* 2009;24(1):3–12

Cartland JD, Yudkowsky BK. Barriers to pediatric referral in managed care systems. *Pediatrics.* 1992;89(2):183–192

Grupp-Phelan J, Delgado SV, Kelleher KJ. Failure of psychiatric referrals from the pediatric emergency department. *BMC Emerg Med.* 2007;7:12

Howard BJ. The referral role of pediatricians. *Pediatr Clin North Am.* 1995;42:103–118

Igelhart JK. Physicians and the growth of managed care. *N Engl J Med.* 1994;331:1167

Kahn RS, Wise PH, Finkelstein JA, et al. The scope of unmet maternal health needs in pediatric settings. *Pediatrics.* 1999;103:576–581

Krugman SD, Wissow LS. Helping children with troubled parents. *Pediatr Ann.* 1998;27(1):23–29

Pangburn DA. Referral processes. In: Levine MD, Carey WB, Crocker AC, eds. *Developmental–Behavioral Pediatrics.* 3rd ed. Philadelphia, PA: WB Saunders; 1999

Sarvet B, Gold J, Bostic JQ, et al. Improving access to mental health care for children: the Massachusetts Child Psychiatry Access Program. *Pediatrics.* 2010;126(6):1191–1200

Sarvet BD, Wegner L. Developing effective child psychiatry collaboration with primary care: leadership and management strategies. *Child Adolesc Psychiatr Clin N Am.* 2010;19(1):139–148

Steele MM, Lochrie AS, Roberts MC. Physician identification and management of psychosocial problems in primary care. *J Clin Psychol Med Settings.* 2010;17(2):103–115

Verhulst FC, Ende J. Factors associated with child mental health service use in the community. *J Am Acad Child Adolesc Psychiatr* 1997;36(7):773–777

Correct Use of Procedural and Diagnostic Codes to Document Family-Focused Pediatric Care

Lynn M. Wegner, MD, FAAP

*P*roviding family-centered care likely is a goal of anyone reading this book. Most of us, however, do not practice in a system that readily pays for extended office visits or non–face-to-face work. Family-centered care involves meeting the needs of at least 2 patients—the child and the family—yet the current payment system functions as though meeting these dual needs is no more complicated than making the diagnosis of a viral pharyngeal infection! The current US payment system is poorly understood by anyone except "coding geeks" and regulatory experts, and the medical provider attempting to get paid for providing mental health service. It seems to be a quagmire of poorly understood codes. While most of these codes describe the face-to-face medical services to payers, there is almost always work beyond the office encounter with the family. Throughout this book, there are numerous examples of the pediatric care professional (PCP) talking with a parent, reviewing notes from outside sources and rating scale results, talking with community resources, etc, *before* the face-to-face appointment. There is also work expected *after* the appointment (the summary letter to the family; calls to teachers, therapists, and other family members; and written reports and letters documenting the needs for services). The PCP dealing with patient mental health and family needs is expected to understand how all of this non–face-to-face work interfaces with the procedure code documented on the day of the appointment. The result is that the PCP is expected to absorb all the preservice and post-service work—and be grateful, at that, for any payment. While clinicians may rail against the current payment system, which undervalues cognitive work unaccompanied by procedures, the current system may be used more successfully if the PCP understands the system and appropriately creates clinical services in synchrony with the current payment structure. This does not mean abandoning *quality* care, but it does mean an understanding of *efficient* care.

If the medical provider is in a solo practice, there is both good news and bad news. The good news is that this individual may be responsible for all procedural coding for work done under the practice tax number. This is definite quality control, as the provider knows what was done during the service and, if the provider understands *Current Procedural Terminology (CPT®)*[1] codes, those services can be completely and accurately described through the *CPT* codes. If a provider is located in a tertiary system, the coding professionals or business manager employed may not be cognizant of what is done during the appointment and what the actual services comprise. This ignorance may result in undercoding and resultant underpayment for properly provided and documented medical care! While it may not seem fair, it may very well fall on the shoulders of the PCPs to insist that those individuals responsible for the institutional billing truly understand the complexity, time required, and importance of the mental health services. Not all work need be considered preservice or post-service work. While it is easier for the coders to lump all work into the office encounter, it is not equitable to those PCPs providing these necessary ancillary services.

The outpatient face-to-face codes, pertinent to primary care family-focused mental health services, describe new, established, consultation, and preventive evaluation and management (E/M) services. There are also codes for behavioral and developmental screening and ratings assessment. If a service was modified in some manner, modifiers may be appended to the basic service code to tell the payers that outpatient (and inpatient) services were modified and this change may result in altered payment. Non–face-to-face services are clearly essential to providing family-focused care, and so there are codes for telephone care, online medical evaluation, care plan oversight, extensive reports, and team conferences.

While this chapter cannot be a coding tome for mental health care, it does describe documentation of common services by procedural (*CPT*) codes resulting in efficient payment. Part I describes codes for face-to-face services (E/M), behavioral screening and rating scales, modifier use, and appropriately accounting for extra service time using prolonged service codes. Non–face-to-face service codes for care plan oversight, telephone care, special reports, and electronic messages are found in Part II. Part III explains coding for the most accurate *International Classification of Diseases, Ninth Revision,*

Clinical Modification (ICD-9-CM)[2] diagnosis when use of mental health codes (ie, *Diagnostic and Statistical Manual, Fourth Edition, Text Revision [DSM-IV-TR]*[3] codes **290–319**) results in a payer being carved out as a mental health provider. Part IV describes steps to be taken if payment is denied by third-party payers after proper documentation.

PART I: INITIAL FACE-TO-FACE SERVICES, MODIFIERS, RATING SCALES, AND PROLONGED SERVICES

Face-to-Face Services: Coding for the Initial Visit, With and Without Screening or Rating Scales

The initial visit suggesting the utility of a family-focused visit may occur coincidently during a visit for another medical condition or during an anticipatory guidance visit. Family issues may also be identified by a general psychosocial screening instrument administered to the parent and/or the patient. Outpatient mental health care is provided through E/M services. These services include preventive health care for new (**99381–99384**) and established (**99391–99394**) patients, new (**99201–99205**) and established (**99211–99215**) patient office visits, and consultation (**99241–99245**) services on request by another appropriate professional. In its 2010 Resource-Based Relative Value Scale final rule, the Centers for Medicare & Medicaid Services (CMS) decided to eliminate payment for consultation codes (**99241–99245; 99251–99255**) in the Medicare program effective January 1, 2010. In order to maintain Medicare budget neutrality, the consultation codes' relative values were redistributed to the new and established office visit codes (**99201–99215**) and the initial hospital (**99221–99223**) and nursing facility (**99304–99306**) codes.

A patient may be considered "new" if the provider or any other provider from the same specialty in the same medical group practice either has never provided care or has not seen the patient in the past 3 years. Health supervision (well-child checkups)/preventive medicine visits are properly described by the preventive medicine services for children (new patient **99381**, established patient **99391**: <1 year old; **99382, 99392**: 1–4 years; **99383, 99393**: 5–11 year) and adolescents (**99384, 99394**: 12–17 years) codes (**99384** and **99394**). These codes, like the other E/M codes, are subcategorized as new patient or established patient. Codes in these series are selected based on the age of the patient and not on the basis of time spent on the date of service.

All E/M services, with the exception of preventive visits, may be coded on the basis of either the complexity of the visit or on the amount of time required on the date of service. These same non-preventive E/M visits are defined in 4 levels of service: problem focused, expanded problem focused, detailed problem focused, and comprehensive. Complexity entails consideration of the 3 key components: history recorded, elements of the physical examination performed, and the complexity of the medical decision-making required by the provider. Tables 32.1 and 32.2 illustrate the 5 levels of new and established patient visits, and the face-to-face time expected by *CPT*. Note the times accompanying the code number on the following tables are average values that may be lesser or greater depending on the clinical circumstances of the encounter.

MODIFIERS

Modifiers are 2-digit suffixes appended to the end of a *CPT* code to tell the payer that "this visit was different." The service may have been altered by a specific situation described by the modifier. Some modifiers may only be used with E/M codes, and others only may accompany procedures. Modifier use is extremely important, as they enable the payer software to permit these special circumstances. When modifiers are used, however, the provider must take care to clearly document the circumstances supporting their use. Listing modifiers on the billing sheet will encourage their use! Despite correct modifier use and supportive documentation in the medical record, not all payers recognize and/or pay for all modifiers.

Modifier **25** (significant, separately identifiable E/M service by the same physician on the same day as the procedure or other service) tells the payer that the documentation requirements were met for a separate E/M service or procedure during that visit. Take, for example, a session where the family returned their completed behavioral rating scales and the appointment included a lengthy discussion of current family concerns, efficacy of recommendations made at a previous appointment, and new intervention suggestions. All discussion would contribute to the level of the separate E/M service selected. Modifier **25** would be properly appended to the E/M code to inform the payer that this E/M visit was separate from the scoring and interpretation of the rating scales returned at this visit. The medical record should have 2 separate sections documenting the 2 separate services: a note summarizing the family session and a brief separate note indicating which rating scales were completed and by whom, the results of the scored rating scales, and how this information is going to be used in the management of this family's concerns.

Another example of correct modifier **25** use would be the situation when the parent completes a behavioral screening instrument (eg, Pediatric Symptom Checklist-17[5]) as part of a preventive medical care visit. In that situation, the procedure is described by code **96110** (developmental testing, limited) and modifier **25** would be properly appended to the selected **993xx** code, and **96110** also would be included as a separate service charge. Again, there must

Table 32.1. New Patient Office Visit (expected time/minutes)[a]

Codes	99201 (10)	99202 (20)	99203 (30)	99204 (45)	99205 (60)
History	Problem focused	Expanded problem focused	Detailed	Comprehensive	Comprehensive
Exam	Problem focused	Expanded problem focused	Detailed	Comprehensive	Comprehensive
Decision-making	Straightforward	Straightforward	Low complexity	Moderate complexity	High complexity
Key components[b]	3 of 3	3 of 3	3 of 3	3 of 3	3 of 3

[a]Adapted from American Academy of Pediatrics. Coding for Pediatrics 2010. Elk Grove Village, IL: American Academy of Pediatrics; 2010:52–53.
[b]Key components: history, physical examination, and medical decision-making.

Table 32.2. Established Patient Office Visit (expected time/minutes)[a]

Codes	99211 (5)	99212 (10)	99213 (15)	99214 (25)	99215 (40)
History	Not required	Problem focused	Expanded problem focused	Detailed	Comprehensive
Exam	Not required	Problem focused	Expanded problem focused	Detailed	Comprehensive
Decision-making	Not required	Straightforward	Low complexity	Moderate complexity	High complexity
Key components[b]	2 of 3	2 of 3	2 of 3	2 of 3	2 of 3

[a]Adapted from American Academy of Pediatrics. Coding for Pediatrics 2010. Elk Grove Village, IL: American Academy of Pediatrics; 2010:52–53.
[b]Key components: history, physical examination, and medical decision-making.

be separate sections in the medical record for the 2 provided services and whether or not the 2 services are paid is up to the payer.

Modifier **32** (mandated services) is used when a third party requires the service being provided. For example, if a second opinion of a mental health or behavioral diagnosis is required before a child may receive treatment, modifier **32** would be appended to the E/M code describing the visit providing that evaluation service.

Modifiers used with procedures and not E/M codes include modifier **59** (distinct procedural service). This code is used when procedures not usually reported together do occur appropriately on the same date of service. It indicates the procedure was distinct from the other procedures performed on that same date of service. Coders refer to this modifier as the "modifier of last resort," and the physician should be satisfied that no other modifier would be more appropriate. Clear documentation is always required to support payment of both procedures. An example of the use of modifier **59** would be a second office visit for family counseling and a patient neurobehavioral status examination **(96116),** during which the parents also returned rating scales completed by the patient's child care provider for scoring and interpretation **(96110)**. Modifier **59** would be appended to the second procedure marked on the billing sheet.

Modifier **76** (repeat procedure by the same physician or other qualified health professional) is appended when a physician or other qualified health provider performs the same procedure more than once, and use of this code tells the payer the repeated procedure is not a duplicate service. (This modifier should not be appended to an E/M service.) The procedure may be repeated on different dates of service, and modifier **76** is appended to the procedure code. Documentation must identify each separate procedure. For example, if 3 Vanderbilt attention-deficit/hyperactivity disorder (ADHD) scales[6] (mother, teacher, and custodial father in a divorced family) are completed, scored, and interpreted in conjunction with a **99215** E/M visit, then those 3 (**96110**: developmental testing, limited) procedures could be coded as

99215-25
96110
96110-76
96110-76

Another way of coding multiple units of the same rating scale in the above example would be

99215-25
(3) 96110

If the payer refuses use of modifier **76** for the **96110** codes or the use of a number to describe the multiple units of **96110,** the visit could be coded as

99215-25

96110-59

96110-59

96110-59

CODING FOR RATING SCALE AND BEHAVIORAL SCREENING INSTRUMENTS

96110 Developmental Testing, Limited: Use for Screening and Behavioral Rating Scales

At the time of the publication of this edition, standardized screening instruments and behavioral/emotional rating scales are documented appropriately using code **96110** (developmental testing, limited), and this code may be listed for as many forms as are completed, scored, and interpreted. For example, if a Pediatric Symptom Checklist-17[5] is given to both parents and scored, 2 units of **96110** may be coded: **(2) 96110.** As there is no "physician work" in the code valuation, the screens would be appropriately administered and scored by a non-primary provider in the office (eg, medical or nursing assistant, receptionist) but reviewed, interpreted, and discussed with the family by the PCP. The results would then be included in the medical record in a brief summary of the result interpretation. (This summary is the "report" included in the *CPT* descriptor for developmental testing, limited: **96110.**) When mental health screening is performed as part of a preventive medicine visit, the basic service (new patient**: 99381–99384**; established patient: **99391–99394**) is documented along with the developmental screening code **(96110).** A modifier is appended to the preventive service code to identify the visit as a separate and identifiable service from the "procedure code"—the developmental testing, limited (aka developmental screening). Some payers may not pay separately for this and may bundle this screening and/or behavioral rating into the preventive service. This separate payment is not a coding issue, but rather a payer issue.

Example of preventive service for a new 12- to 17-year-old patient with 2 behavioral screening instruments (eg, Patient Symptom Checklist-17[5], Patient Health Questionnaire-9[7]) administered, scored, reviewed, discussed, and reported in the medical record note

99384-25

(2) 96110

If the payer does not allow the use of modifier **25,** this visit could alternatively be coded as

99384

96110-59

96110-59

As children enter adolescence, routine well-child visits may not occur
with the regularity with which they occurred in early childhood. For this
reason, many PCPs screen for mental health conditions at visits for reasons
other than preventive health care. Again, the mental health screening instruments may appropriately be given to the parent (adult accompanying the
teen to the visit) and the teen, scored, and then interpreted. Positive endorse-
ments found through the screening can be discussed at that visit, or a subsequent visit can be suggested after the parent and patient are given the results
of the screening. Coding the screening, as discussed earlier, would occur by
appending modifier **25** (separate and identifiable service from the screening
procedure) to the appropriate E/M service and writing on the billing sheet the
number of screening instruments administered, scored, interpreted, and documented. The chosen E/M level of service would properly reflect either the
complexity of the service or the time spent if more than 50% of the visit was
spent in counseling and/or care coordination. If time is the criterion chosen,
it is very helpful to note the time the visit began, the time it concluded, the
amount of time spent in counseling, and documentation of the counseling
elements discussed.

Example of a 15-minute face-to-face urgent-care visit for allergic rhinitis
for an established patient with 2 screening instruments administered, scored,
reviewed, discussed, and reported in the medical record

99213-25

(2) 96110

ICD-9: 477.0

V40.9 Unspecified mental or behavioral problem

While less common, it is possible that a new patient will arrive in your
office specifically for a behavioral/mental health concern and not a preventive
services visit (patient office visit: **99201–99205**). Again, if screening tools are
used, they should be coded in addition with **96110** and the modifier **25** added
to the codes **99202–99205** or modifier **59** added to the procedure code(s).

FOLLOW-UP VISITS AFTER EITHER A POSITIVE SCREEN INSTRUMENT OR IDENTIFICATION OF FAMILY ISSUES

If the patient and/or parent agrees to a subsequent visit to discuss the family
concerns identified through screening at the initial non–mental health visit,
the follow-up visit ideally should be allotted more time than a standard visit

for a physical problem. If a practice customarily schedules 5 patients an hour (12 minutes/visit), then 2 slots should be given for the family-focused follow-up visit. Ideally, this visit might occur at the end of an office day so more time could be spent if significant and more time-requiring issues emerge. It will be important for the PCP to remember that the basis for coding any established E/M visit is based on either complexity of service or time spent with the child and/or family. If 50% of the visit was spent in counseling and/or care coordination, time must be used as the factor for code level selection. The documentation requirements are noted in Table 32.2. If complexity is used, however, there must be documentation for 2 out of 3 elements of history, physical examination, or medical decision-making, even at the minimally complex level. Considering the reason for the follow-up visit is a mental health concern, it is unlikely this visit would be focused on either history or physical examination; it most likely involved counseling and/or coordination of mental health services. Time would be the most appropriate and logical criterion on which to base the visit charge. Time-based coding does seem most appropriate and the best established E/M code for this example of a "2 slot" 24-minute appointment and would be **99214** (24 minutes face-to-face time). Twenty-four minutes is more than halfway between the 15 minutes required for **99213** and 25 minutes needed for **99214.** For that reason, the higher level code is chosen. A notation would need to be included in the medical record that the visit lasted 24 minutes and documentation must specify that 13 minutes or more (>50% of the visit) were devoted to "counseling and/or coordination of care." Documentation requirements for a time-based visit also must include a summary of this "counseling and/or care coordination."

Example of Counseling Documentation

The Vanderbilt ADHD Scales–Teacher Version was completed by John's teacher, Ms Susan Jones. Her responses yielded 2/9 "often" statements for the inattention statements (1–9) and 3/9 "often" statements for the hyperactivity questions (10–18). No functional impairment statements were scored greater than 2, indicating she did not see impairment in his classroom performance. Fifteen minutes was then spent discussing the lack of functional impairment at school, while his mother's responses on the Vanderbilt scales at the previous visit were significantly "positive" (9/9) for her observations of John's difficulty with inattention and hyperactivity at home and in the community outside of school. John's mother feels his behavior has deteriorated over the past 6 months. When I asked about any new changes at home, she admitted she and John's father have been worried about their income. John's father now has 2 jobs and John's mother is taking in ironing and providing after-school care for 2 neighbor children. John has had to stop his tae kwon do classes and his bicycle is broken.

John, his mother, and I discussed ways of expending extra energy after school. His mother reassured him that although money is short now, his father's primary job is secure and she doesn't mind the extra work. I encouraged increasing his attendance at an after-school activities program, working on more regular bedtime practices, and encouraging daily jogging through their neighborhood with an older brother. A mood diary was given and explained. By the end of the 25-minute visit, John agreed with the plans, responded without rancor to several comments directed at him by his mother, and agreed to meet in 2 weeks for an update on his progress. We made no medication changes.

PROLONGED SERVICES

Medical visits for discerning, discussing, developing, and modifying management plans for family concerns identified at other appointments obviously can exceed the customary time slots in a pediatric primary care setting. To permit extended time for the often complex and detailed discussions with a family that may be confronting mental health issues for the first time, appointments might best be scheduled at the end of the day. The PCP needs to remember the highest level time code for an established patient is 40 minutes of face-to-face time. If the appointment exceeds 40 minutes, then the *CPT* system has codes permitting documentation for "prolonged services." As mentioned previously, while prolonged services codes are usually used in conjunction with the higher level E/M codes, they may correctly be used for lower levels of service when complexity is the code selection criterion. Prolonged services codes allow reporting both face-to-face and non–face-to-face time with patients and, while these codes must be appropriately selected for the factor of direct contact, the time does not have to be continuous. All prolonged time *on the same day of service* may be combined for the total time reported (Table 32.3).

To correctly account for prolonged time beyond that specified in the selected E/M code, the first 30 minutes exceeding the E/M time is still included in the initial E/M payment. (This is considered customary post-service work.) Therefore, a prolonged service code may not be used until after the first 30 minutes of the prolonged services has been provided. The medical provider has to spend 31 to 74 minutes with the patient and/or family in prolonged services before it is possible to correctly code for 31 minutes using code **99354.** What if the total prolonged services exceed 74 minutes? Code **99355** applies for each additional 30 minutes spent in face-to-face contact beyond the initial prolonged face-to–face 74 service minutes. To correctly use **99355,** however, the medical provider must spend at least 15 minutes beyond the initial 74 minutes of prolonged time.

Table 32.3. Time Guidelines for Prolonged Outpatient E/M Services (99354–99359)	
Total Duration of Prolonged Services	**Codes**
Face to face <30 minutes	Not reported separately
Face to face, 30–74 minutes	**99354**
Face to face, 75–104 minutes	**99355,** each additional 30 minutes, past 74 minutes, use with **99354**
Face to face, 105–134 minutes	**99354** x 1 plus **99355** x 2
Before or after face to face, <30 minutes	Not reported separately
Before or after face to face, 30–74 minutes	**99358**
Before or after face to face, 75–104 minutes	**99359,** each additional 30 minute, past 74 minutes, use with **99358**
Before or after face to face, 105–134 minutes	**99358** x 1 plus **99359** x 2

Example of Coding Prolonged Services

Mary, a 10-year-old established patient, whose mother recently returned to the home after a 6-month incarceration for shoplifting, is seen for monitoring of her ADHD by her PCP. The diagnosis was made after her mother began her sentence. Mary's mother is in a transition work program, therefore the visit was scheduled at the end of the clinic day. For the past 2 months Mary has been receiving behavioral therapy from a community psychologist. Mary's mother not only has many additional—and quite different—observations of her daughter's demeanor as a little child, but also has very definite opinions about her daughter's ADHD diagnosis and treatment plan, and the appropriateness of the combined treatment plan prescribed for Mary. The entire appointment lasts 125 minutes, not including a 10-minute break for the medical provider to take a telephone call from the child's therapist.

Time is used as the appointment code selection criterion.

99215 (established patient, outpatient visit; 40 minutes' duration)

99354 (prolonged services, first 30–74 minutes beyond the 30 minutes post-visit)

If the total face-to-face visit lasted 144 minutes

99215 (established patient, outpatient visit; 40 minutes' duration)

99354 (prolonged services, first 30–74 minutes beyond the 30 minutes post-visit)

99355 x 1 (prolonged services, each 30 minutes beyond the first 60 minutes post-appointment)

PART II: NON–FACE-TO-FACE SERVICES AS PART OF CASE MANAGEMENT

Care Plan Oversight

It is clear from the clinical examples provided throughout this book that PCPs often collaborate, coordinate, and share care with "virtual teams" of community-based mental health specialists to create comprehensive care plans for their families. This is especially true for PCPs who may refer their patients for additional supportive services or their patients' parents to ancillary providers. Services related to acquiring additional information about the patient's ongoing condition and provided without the patient or family present are generally referred to as *case management services*. Telephone calls, team conferences, written reports, and care plan oversight for children and teens living at home and in group homes all fall in the case management realm. Unfortunately, these services do not automatically and uniformly result in payment to the PCP.

If the patient is taking medication prescribed by a child psychiatrist, the PCP may provide monitoring of the medication efficacy and side effects at medical visits for non–mental health reasons in between periodic medication follow-up appointments with the psychiatrist. If the child psychiatrist is located a significant distance from the child's home, the PCP may even serve as the primary professional monitoring and adjusting the medication while consulting with the child psychiatrist by telephone. Other professionals may also serve roles in the virtual team. The patient's individual psychotherapist; teacher(s); coaches; and/or speech/language, occupational, or physical therapists may have important observations of the child's status. The PCP may regularly talk with these individuals and use this information in managing the child's care plan and/or the family's counseling. This supervision of the child's management and family progress requires time, obtaining ongoing history from multiple sources and frequent complex medical decision-making. For this regular non–face-to-face information collection and plan modification, there are care plan oversight codes **99338** (15–29 minutes/month) and **99339** (>29 minutes/month): recurrent physician supervision of a complex patient or a patient who requires multidisciplinary care and ongoing physician involvement. These non–face-to-face services are reported separately from E/M services by the physician who has the supervisory role in the patient's care or is the sole provider. Both **99338** and **99339** reflect the complexity and time required to supervise the care of the patient and are reported based on the amount of time spent in a calendar month. Tasks appropriately included in this service would include reviewing laboratory results as part of medication monitoring; assessing a patient's progress in related but non-psychotherapeutic therapies (eg, speech/language, occupational, or physical therapies); and documenting behavioral changes in family dynamics and interactions through telephone calls or written communication with other professionals frequently interacting and observing the family. These codes are reported only once monthly and reflect the total time spent by the primary provider as care manager. To ensure accuracy in time calculation, a care log in which time and services are recorded can be very helpful (Table 32.4). A copy of this log can be attached when the billing sheet is submitted to the insurer if there are denials for this service.

Telephone Care (99371–99373)

The clinical examples provided throughout this book illustrate the important role of telephone care in working with families. Communication between the PCP and therapists, teachers, school counselors, and family members can be important to optimal management. There are 3 published telephone care codes for physician telephone calls (**99441–99443**), and relative value units (RVUs) have been assigned to them (**9944x:** telephone E/M service initiated by the patient, provided by a physician to an established patient, parent, or guardian not originating from a related E/M service provided within the previous 7 days nor leading to an E/M service or procedure within the next 24 hours or soonest available appointment). See Table 32.5.

While telephone calls to non–family members may be included in care management services, and therefore cannot be submitted for payment if care plan oversight codes have been used, telephone calls by the physician to the child's family can be appropriately billed as a separate and justifiable service in addition to care plan oversight if the requirements for telephone care as a separate service are met. It is very important to determine if the telephone care is more properly classified as preservice or post-service work to the face-to-face office visit.

The American Academy of Pediatrics (AAP) policy statement "Payment for Telephone Care"[8] advocates payment by insurers for correctly documented telephone care. The AAP encourages PCPs to develop policies for their practices, communicate these policies to families, and submit bills for telephone care.

Electronic Communications: Online E/M Service (99244)

More and more, older children, teens, adults, and even PCPs routinely use electronic messaging to communicate quickly. Using electronic means (Internet or other electronic means) to communicate with patients and families is a decision each PCP must make, and this decision reflects many factors. There is, however, a *CPT* code permitting documentation of this service for payment request (**99444:** online E/M by a physician). While few payers are remitting payment for this service as RVUs have not yet been assigned,

Table 32.4. Example of Service and Time Log for Care Management by Pediatric Care Professional

Date Last Face-to-Face Visit	Service	Date of Service	Action	Time for Service (minutes)	Cumulative Time for Month
9/15/10	Telephone call to child psychiatrist	10/1/10	Discussed current fluoxetine dose	10	10
9/15/10	Telephone call w/ lead school teacher	10/2/10	Discussed more convenient time for parent/teacher conference	5	15
9/15/10	Telephone call w/ guidance counselor	10/6/10	Discussed modifying IEP	10	25
9/15/10	Telephone call w/mother	10/18/10	Discussed patient's refusal to participate in 'game night'	10	35
9/15/10	Review of rating scales	10/21/10	Reviewed teacher and speech pathologist Vanderbilt Scales: appointment needed to discuss modifying stimulant dose	12	47 minutes total

Table 32.5. Telephone Care by a Physician to the Patient/Family (99441–99443)

Code	Time, min	Level of Work	Example
99441	5–10	Simple or brief	Report on tests; clarify instructions; adjust treatment
99442	11–20	Intermediate	Advice on problem; start treatment; discuss tests results in detail
99443	21–30	Complex	Lengthy counseling; prolonged discussion on serious condition

the code has been approved by the CMS. There are expectations, however, with the code: a physician provides this service, the patient or the family of the patient initiates the electronic contact, the service is rendered to an established patient, and the communication is not related to an E/M service provided within the previous 7 days. If electronic communication is used, there are some important practical liability considerations. First, the decision must be made if communication will be made only with a patient or families who had a face-to-face contact. Professionals who give advice on the Internet may be creating a duty to a patient—even if the patient has never been seen as a patient! This duty is not dependent on whether or not payment is collected or if the advice was solicited. Second, e-mail creates a written, reproducible, signed, and dated document accessible to the patient. It creates a document that may be admissible in a court of law. If the decision is made to permit electronic communication to facilitate patient care, financial decisions must be made. If the payer does not pay for e-mails, and the physician desires payment for this service, then policies similar to those suggested for telephone care should be considered. Alerting families of their need to pay for electronic messages should be done before a bill requesting payment is sent to them.

Team Conferences (99367)

Sometimes the virtual team meets in person to discuss the patient's status. It is assumed that all participants are actively involved in the decision-making about the continued care and plan development for the patient. Moreover, the PCP should have performed face-to-face evaluations or treatments within the prior 60 days. To correctly submit a code for payment for a physician participating in a multidisciplinary team conference, the following expectation must be met: There must be face-to-face participation by a minimum of 3 qualified health professionals from different disciplines who are all providing direct care to the patient. The patient, family members, or any concerned individual adult need **not** be present at the meeting. This code assumes the PCP has reviewed materials prior to the meeting, and this code covers any post-meeting documentation of PCP participation in the meeting, revised treatment recommendations, and revised review of the care plan for the teen. Therefore, if the PCP submits a bill for participation in this meeting this work should not be included in the time underlying any care plan oversight payment request.

Special Reports/Form Completion

While parents may purchase insurance covering mental health care for their children, insurers may require extensive documentation of the need for this care on special forms. Self-contained schools and camps for children with significant physical and/or mental health conditions may require the PCP to complete extensive forms for the child's admission. Procedure code **99080** (special reports such as insurance forms, more than the information conveyed in the usual medical communication or standard reporting form) is published and may be used for these services. There are no RVUs assigned to this code, however, and payers may not pay for this service. Clinicians should develop an office policy, similar to the decision for billing for telephone care, and advise families in advance if they will be expected to pay for this service.

PART III: *ICD-9-CM* CODING

The *ICD-9-CM* contains all of the labels for services provided in health care: the "reason" for the encounter. Mental health conditions are found between *ICD-9-CM* numbers **290–319,** and these conditions comprise the codes listed in the *DSM-IV-TR*. Unfortunately, not all the names of the diagnoses in the *DSM-IV-TR* map clearly onto the *ICD-9-CM* names, and some insurance providers require *ICD-9-CM* codes and not *DSM-IV-TR* codes. Sometimes the numbers for specific *DSM-IV-TR* conditions are the same as the *ICD-9-CM* codes, but the title of the disorder is different. The American Psychological Association Practice Organization has designed a crosswalk, a document to help determine which *ICD-9-CM* diagnosis code corresponds to a *DSM-IV-TR* diagnosis code (www.apapractice.org).

The clinician should code the diagnosis to the highest level of diagnostic *certainty* (the words in the descriptor) and *complexity* (the numbers in the *ICD-9-CM* codes.) The first diagnosis listed on the billing sheet, however, should be the condition being actively managed on that date of service. A chronic condition, such as ADHD or depression, managed on an ongoing basis may be coded and reported as many times as applicable to the patient's treatment. There is no provision for "rule out" in *ICD-9-CM* , but there is a code (**799.99,** deferred diagnosis). This could be properly used, however, payers may not choose to pay if **799.99** is listed first.

On the billing sheet, the first code selected is the condition the physician is actively managing during the visit ("the reason for the visit"). Subsequently documented codes identify factors important to the primary condition and coexisting conditions being managed/treated along with the primary condition. If a child is seen for a residual condition (eg, **313.83,** academic underachievement disorder), code this first with the cause of the condition as a secondary *ICD-9-CM* code (eg, **331.83**, mild cognitive impairment, so stated).

It is extremely important to understand that the diagnostic code does not determine the level of complexity of the service code. Any diagnosis can support varying levels of service. It is quite possible ADHD could support a *CPT* level 3 code as well as a level 5 code. See Table 32.6.

Table 32.6. Other *ICD-9-CM* Codes Describing Developmental/Behavioral Conditions, Not Including 290–319

DSM-IV-TR Code	*DSM-IV-TR* Title	*ICD-9-CM* Code	*ICD-9-CM* Title
314.01	Attention-deficit disorder, with mention of hyperactivity, combined subtype	799.51	Attention or concentration deficit (not associated with attention deficit disorder): Use before diagnosis is made.
314.00	Attention-deficit disorder, without mention of hyperactivity, predominately inattentive subtype	799.55	Frontal lobe and executive function deficit
315.4	Developmental coordination disorder	781.3	Lack of coordination
307.9	Communication disorder, not otherwise specified	783.42	Late talking or late walking
299.0	Autism	799.52	Cognitive communication deficit
315.02	Developmental dyslexia	784.61	Alexia and dyslexia

Abbreviations: *DSM-IV-TR, Diagnostic and Statistical Manual, Fourth Edition, Text Revision; ICD-9-CM, International Classification of Diseases, Ninth Revision, Clinical Modification.*

There are V codes in the *ICD-9-CM* terminology. These codes, variably paid by insurers, are used to deal with occasions when circumstances other than a disease or injury are recorded as "diagnoses" or "problems." For example, a V code may be used when a patient who is not currently sick encounters a health provider for some specific service (eg, weight or blood pressure check for medication monitoring). V codes also may properly be used when a patient presents for a specific treatment of a known condition or disease. V codes also may be used when a patient's health status is influenced by some circumstance that is not in itself a current injury or illness (eg, parental history of alcoholism). See Table 32.7.

PART IV: REASONS FOR DENIAL OF COVERAGE DESPITE PROPER DOCUMENTATION

If all of the above instructions are followed and the coverage is denied, then the patient's particular policy may not cover the service in question or the diagnosis. For example, some insurance providers will not pay for physician

Table 32.7. Family Concerns V Codes (Not Inclusive)			
V61.20	Counseling for parent-child problem, unspecified	**V60.89**	Other specified housing or family circumstances
V61.29	Parent-child problems, other	**V40.2**	Other mental problems
V65.49	Other specified counseling	**V 40.3**	Mental and behavioral problems; other behavioral problems
V65.5	Person with feared complaint in whom no diagnosis was made	**V 40.9**	Unspecified mental or behavioral problem
V65.8	Other reasons for seeking consultation	**V 69.8**	Other problems related to lifestyle
V62.81	Interpersonal problems, not elsewhere classified	**V61.0**	Family disruption

phone calls around mental health even if coded properly (**99441–99443**). In other words, if a family functioning assessment is a phone follow-up and not a face-to-face visit, the PCP may not be paid even with proper documentation. In addition, in cases where there are behavioral health carve-outs, a PCP who codes a visit with a depression or anxiety diagnosis may be refused payment by the primary care portion of the plan. When coverage is denied, the first thing to do is inspect the billing sheet for errors in accurately placing *CPT* or *ICD-9-CM* numbers for accurate identification of the service provided and the reason supporting the service. If this is correct, then the parent/guardian may need to read their contract with the insurer to see if the service was, in fact, promised as part of the contract. Every patient/guardian should read their contract with the payer. Although the verbiage may be obtuse, the services covered are listed in this document. It is very unfortunate, but many patients (or their parents/guardians) do not understand the language of these legal documents. Many patients do not have a choice regarding their health care coverage. For those who can choose, cost is often in their foremost thoughts. Unfortunately, mental health coverage is often carefully written into the contract and the exclusions often are not uncovered until the need is there. Certain practices will be able to charge patients directly for services not covered by their insurance plans. Those practices should also enlist these self-pay families to join grassroots efforts to make mental health parity a reality and not just a piece of legislation. When enough families complain about poor mental health coverage, policy will change. Some families may be able to switch their coverage, and PCPs can encourage families to look into this option. Other practices will have to accept temporarily that their services will not be paid. In certain cases, the practice manager or the PCP should try to renegotiate their contracts with the insurance carrier so that these services are covered in the future. Sometimes joining with other practices in the area or the state or with the local or regional chapters of professional organizations (such as the councils of the state AAP chapters) can give more clout to such renegotiation. Mental health screening should be thought of just like vaccines for infectious diseases: a routine clinical necessity with spotty payment coverage that has since sparked advocacy and solutions.

Summary

Pediatric care professionals can have an important role in helping their patients enjoy optimal mental health. Understanding efficient methods of care and modifying practice habits to minimize services not currently supported by procedural codes and better documenting those covered services will permit the PCP to be paid for this medical care. Current medical procedure codes can be legitimately used to bill for family-focused care, and consistent use of these codes will help address payment barriers. As more PCPs enthusiastically participate in the management of their patients' family issues, the medical home will provide more complete health care.

This coding content was accurate as of March 9, 2011. CPT © 2011 American Medical Association (AMA). All rights reserved. The AMA assumes no liability for data contained herein. CPT is a registered trademark of the AMA.

References

1. American Medical Association. *Current Procedural Terminology*. Chicago, IL: American Medical Association Press; 2010
2. Chrisendres.com *Free Online Searchable ICD 2009 ICD-9 CM*. http://icd9cm.chrisendres.com Accessed January 10, 2011
3. American Psychiatric Association. *Diagnostic and Statistical Manual-Fourth Edition—Text Revision*. Arlington, VA: American Psychiatric Press; 2000
4. American Academy of Pediatrics. *Coding for Pediatrics Coding 2010*. Elk Grove Village, IL: American Academy of Pediatrics; 2010
5. *Pediatric Symptom Checklist-17*. www2.massgeneral.org/allpsych/psc/psc_forms.htm
6. Vanderbilt ADHD Rating Scales. http://able-differently.org/PDF_forms/handouts/ NICHQVanderbiltParent.pdf
7. *Patient Health Questionniare-9*. www.commonwealthfund.org/usr_doc/PHQ-9.pdf
8. American Academy of Pediatrics Section on Telephone Care and Committee on Child Health Financing. Payment for telephone care. *Pediatrics*. 2006;118:1768–1773

Additional Resources

Commercial Pediatric Coding Newsletters

American Academy of Pediatrics. *Pediatric Coding Companion.* Elk Grove Village, IL: American Academy of Pediatrics

The Coding Institute. *Pediatric Coding Alert.* Durham, NC: Eli Research

Web Sites

www.aacap.org
Web site of the American Academy of Child and Adolescent Psychiatry with coding information specific to mental and behavioral health care for children

www.dbpeds.org
Web site of the American Academy of Pediatrics Section on Developmental and Behavioral Pediatrics with coding information specific to developmental and behavioral health care for children

www.apapractice.org
Web site with the American Psychological Association Practice Organization's crosswalk: a document to help determine which *ICD-9-CM* diagnosis code corresponds to a *DSM-IV-TR* diagnosis code

www.cms.hhs.gov/MLNProducts
Documentation guideline revisions by Centers for Medicare & Medicaid Services and the American Medical Association

www.coding.aap.org
American Academy of Pediatrics updates on procedural and diagnostic coding

www.thecodinginstitute.com
Commercial site for coding information

www.schoolpsychiatry.org
Web site developed by Massachusetts General Hospital Division of Psychiatry with extensive information about and links to public domain and proprietary behavioral and emotional rating scales and screening instruments

Glossary

*T*he clinician often encounters new words and terms in the family counseling/therapy literature. Below are definitions of some common words and terms.

Accommodation: The adjustment required by a family or subsystems to coordinate and maintain optimal functioning.

Adaptation: The ability of the family to adapt to alternative interaction patterns in the face of internal or external stress and change. Poor adaptability is a common source of family dysfunction.

Alliance: A healthy, positive relationship between any 2 members of a family (eg, the parents working together or 2 siblings forming a good relationship).

Blended families or stepfamilies: Separate families joined by marriage.

Boundaries: The rules that govern who participates in a subsystem and how they participate. Boundaries protect the integrity and identity of the subsystems. For example, the marital subsystem (husband–wife unit) normally is distinguished from a parent–child subsystem by a boundary (set of rules). Subsystems must be clear and strong enough to prevent a breakdown but flexible enough to provide contact and communication. Assessing boundary clarity and integrity is an essential part of working with families.

Coalition: A relationship among at least 3 persons in which 2 collude or join against a third (eg, a parent and child taking sides against the other parent or a clinician joining with the patient [child] against another family member).

Concurrent therapy: Individual treatment of 2 or more persons usually by different therapists. The physician might see the family, and a marital therapist might see the parents.

Conflict avoidance: When family members do not openly disagree, but allow silent tension and unexpressed needs (covert disagreement) to impact the family negatively. Members may avoid conflict by working harder, by spending more time at their careers or jobs, by interacting less with other members, or by invoking unspoken family "rules."

Conjoint therapy: Treatment of 2 or more persons together in a session.

Cross-generational coalition: An inappropriate or harmful coalition between a parent and a child against a third member of the family. For example, a mother and child may form a coalition against the father.

Cohesion: The amount of closeness (or lack of closeness) in the family relationships.

Contingency contracting: A behavioral therapy technique in which family members agree to exchange rewards for desired behaviors.

Disengagement: Psychological isolation. This term implies that the boundary is too rigid between a subsystem and an individual or between 2 individuals. Members are emotionally distant and unresponsive to each other. For example, if the parent dyad is distant and disengaged with the children, children receive little protection, affection, or support.

Enmeshment: Loss of autonomy due to a blurring of the boundaries. The term implies that the boundary is poorly defined. The family has few or no interpersonal boundaries and little individual autonomy. For example, the marital subsystem has no intimacy/privacy from the children, or a parent may answer questions for a teenager. If little differentiation exists between the parent subsystem and the children, the parental authority is diminished. Enmeshment can also cause family members to be overly involved in each other's feelings and activities; therefore, parents overreact to stress experienced by a child, or a child can overreact to stress experienced by a parent.

Extended families: All the descendants of a set of grandparents.

Family homeostasis: The tendency of families to resist change in order to maintain their steady state or balance; a balanced steady state of equilibrium and family functioning.

Family life cycle: The predictable stages of family life, including leaving home, marriage, birth of children, raising children, growing older, retirement, and death.

Family structure: The functional organization of families that determines members' relationships and how they interact.

Family hierarchy: Family functioning based on a power structure where parents maintain control and authority.

Family interaction patterns: The rules and behaviors that families develop to maintain their stability and structure. These repeating interaction patterns are often passed from generation to generation.

Homeostasis: *See* Family homeostasis.

Identified patient: The symptom bearer or the symptomatic patient of a disturbed family system. The presenting patient as identified by the family (eg, the child who presents with depression in a family with domestic violence).

Joining: The act of the clinician accepting and accommodating to families in order to gain their trust and to circumvent resistance. Part of forming the therapeutic alliance with a family.

Modeling: Observational learning. The parent demonstrates a desirable behavior as a way to teach the child. The clinician may also model desirable behavior as a way to teach the parents.

Nuclear family: The parents and their children.

Overprotectiveness: This occurs when family members are not allowed to deal with their own problems or when parents are too fearful of the possibility that their child might experience an unpleasant event. For example, a mother may refuse to let her child play with other children for fear that he will get hurt.

Parentified child: A child who has been given parent-like power and responsibility to care for a sibling. This phenomenon is adaptive when done deliberately in a large family or single-parent home. It is maladaptive when it stems from unplanned abdication of parent responsibility or when the child "parents" the parent. For example, a depressed single parent may depend on the child to cook the meals, clean the house, and provide comfort to the parent.

Process/content: *Process:* How family members interact and communicate. *Content:* What members communicate about.

Reframing: Relabeling a family's description or perception of a behavior to make the family more accepting of a different explanation or amenable to change (eg, describing a child's temperament/behavior as "strong willed" instead of "oppositional").

Reinforcement: An event, action, or object that increases the recurrence of a particular response. A positive reinforcer is an event or object whose contingent presentation increases the rate of responding. A negative reinforcer is an event or object whose contingent withdrawal increases the rate of responding, whereas a negative consequence is a contingent presentation that decreases the rate of responding.

Rigidity: Family interaction patterns are repeated inflexibly; change is discouraged and resisted.

Subsystems: Smaller units in families determined by generation, gender, or function (eg, the parental [mother–father] unit, the spousal [husband–wife] unit, the parent–child unit, the siblings, or an individual in the family). Subsystems help families carry out their various roles of mutual support, regulation, and socialization. For example, the parent subsystem nurtures and socializes the children; the spousal subsystem provides adult mutual support.

Transference/countertransference: *Transference:* The patient's distorted emotional reaction to a present relationship (including with the physician) that stems from early family relationships. *Countertransference:* The physician's emotional (often unconscious) reaction to the patient or a family member.

Triangulation: A relationship in which a third person is drawn into a 2-person system to diffuse worry or to avoid conflict about personal issues (eg, intimacy) between the 2 persons. For example, a mother and father focus on and argue about their son's behavior instead of confronting their own marital tensions.

Index

Index